M000035658

Children and
Traumatic Incident Reduction
Creative and Cognitive Approaches

Edited by Marian K. Volkman, CTS, CMF

THE TIR APPLICATIONS SERIES

Children and Traumatic Incident Reduction: Creative and Cognitive Approaches
Book number two of the TIR Applications Series
Copyright © 2007 Marian K. Volkman

No part of this publication reproduced, transmitted in any form or by any means, electronic, mechanical, photocopying, recording, or other otherwise, or stored in a retrieval system, without the prior written consent of the publisher.

First Edition: April 2007
Second Printing: March 2010

Library of Congress Cataloging-in-Publication Data

Children and traumatic incident reduction : creative and cognitive approaches / edited by Marian K. Volkman. -- 1st ed.
    p. cm. -- (TIR applications series ; no. 2)
  Includes bibliographical references and index.
  ISBN-13: 978-1-932690-30-9 (trade paper : alk. paper)
  ISBN-10: 1-932690-30-1 (trade paper : alk. paper)
 1. Post-traumatic stress disorder in children--Treatment. 2. Psychic trauma in children--Treatment. 3. Art therapy for children. 4. Cognitive therapy for children. I. Volkman, Marian K. II. Series.
  [DNLM: 1. Stress Disorders, Post-Traumatic--therapy. 2. Art Therapy. 3. Cognitive Therapy. 4. Adolescent. 5. Child. WM 170 C5344 2007]
  RJ506.P55C45 2007
  618.92'8521--dc22
                                        2006030776

Distributed by:
Baker & Taylor, Ingram Book Group,

Published by:
Loving Healing Press
5145 Pontiac Trail
Ann Arbor, MI 48105
USA

http://www.LovingHealing.com or
info@LovingHealing.com
Toll free 888-761-6268
Fax +1 734 663 6861

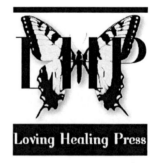

Loving Healing Press

Loving Healing Press

TIR Applications Series

- Traumatic Incident Reduction and Critical Incident Stress Management: A Synergistic Approach
- Children and Traumatic Incident Reduction: Creative and Cognitive Approaches
- Addiction and Traumatic Incident Reduction: A Person-Centered Approach

This new series from Loving Healing Press brings you information and anecdotes about Traumatic Incident Reduction and related techniques used with clients by practitioners around the world. Stories of real-world experience convey the opportunity for healing that TIR provides. Readers interested in the theories behind TIR and Applied Metapsychology (the subject from which TIR is derived) should also consider the *Explorations in Metapsychology* Series from Loving Healing Press. Information about all titles can be found at *www.tirbook.com*

About our Series Editor, Robert Rich, Ph.D.

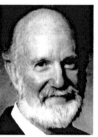

Loving Healing Press is pleased to announce Robert Rich, Ph.D. as Series Editor for the *TIR Applications Series*. This exciting series demonstrates the impacts of TIR and Metapsychology in the real world.

Robert Rich, M.Sc., Ph.D., M.A.P.S., A.A.S.H. is a highly experienced counseling psychologist. His web site *anxietyanddepression-help.com* is a storehouse of helpful information for people suffering from anxiety and depression.

Bob is also a multiple award-winning writer of both fiction and non-fiction, and a professional editor. His writing is displayed at www.bobswriting.com. You are advised not to visit him there unless you have the time to get lost for a while.

Three of his books are tools for psychological self-help: *Anger and Anxiety: Be in charge of your emotions and control phobias, Personally Speaking: Single session email therapy,* and *Cancer: A personal challenge.* However, his philosophy and psychological knowledge come through in all his writing, which is perhaps why three of his books have won international awards, and he has won many minor prizes. Dr. Rich currently resides at Wombat Hollow in Australia.

Table of Contents

Quick Reference to Techniques

Table of Figures

Acknowledgments

Great thanks go to our contributors for sharing their work and stories of their clients with us. In alphabetical order, they are: Janet Buell, Renee Carmody, Tony DeMaria, Teresa Descilo, Anna Foley, Alex Frater, Patricia Furze, Frank A. Gerbode, MD, Brian Grimes, Jessica Hamblen, Jessica Hand, Hildegard Jahn, James Logan, Bob Rich, and Victor Volkman. Many people gave very generously of their time and attention to make this book possible.

A special thank you goes out to Victim Services Miami for allowing us to incorporate materials from their training manual. Also, Renee Carmody, Anna Foley and Patricia Furze were especially generous with their time and each contributed more than one article to this volume.

Appreciation also goes to the young clients who have allowed their stories to be told. Many gave their express and enthusiastic permission. In all cases, the children's names and other identifying information have been changed.

Thanks also to Victor Volkman of Loving Healing Press for permission to reprint the material relating to children from Chapters 1 and 9 from his book, *Beyond Trauma: Conversations on Traumatic Incident Reduction, 2nd Ed* (2005).

Several of the stories and articles in this book appeared in the *Applied Metapsychology International /Traumatic Incident Reduction Association Newsletter* Vols. II and III (ISSN 1555-0818) and are used with permission.

Finally, thanks to you, the reader, for taking an interest in this body of work.

How to Get the Most from this Book

An Introduction to TIR and Children

You will see as you explore this volume that the various writers come from a wide variety of backgrounds in terms of education, experience and mode of practice. Some are individuals in private practice, others work in large agencies. Some are trained and experienced in other methods and use TIR in combination with those methods, while others use TIR and related techniques almost exclusively. A more striking difference, though, is the variety of beliefs and attitudes that is reflected in the writers of these chapters. You may find yourself agreeing with one contributor more than with another.

What brings this group together is their common experience in using Traumatic Incident Reduction (TIR) and related techniques with both children and adults and getting good, rewarding results.

Whether you browse around in this book and read what interests you most, or read it straight through, you will find a rich variety of ideas and techniques. For browsing suggestions, if you work in a hospital setting you will want to look at Chapter 13. If you are a parent and are looking for support for your child, Chapters 6 and 12 will be of special interest. If you like to explore the philosophical structure that underlies a subject, Chapter 14 will be of use. Essential background on the etiology and symptoms of PTSD in children can be found in Chapter 15. At the end, we hope you'll feel compelled to read more case studies and research reports on TIR (see Appendix C).

We have tried to make each chapter as readable as possible as a stand-alone article. In aid of that, you will find a glossary just ahead of the Appendices that defines words specific to the subjects of TIR and Applied Metapsychology. All of the notes and references for each chapter are together, just after the Appendices and before the Index.

Here follows a brief outline of the context of these subjects that will give you a clearer understanding of the chapters ahead.

Frank Gerbode, M.D., the developer of TIR and Applied Metapsychology, has chosen the neutral term, *facilitator* to refer to a practitioner of the subject, rather than "therapist" or "counselor" for the reason that "therapy" can imply that there is something wrong with the person who is coming for help, and "to counsel" means "to advise". Neither of these fits well with the concept of person-centered work. In addition to this, some TIR practitioners are in fact licensed therapists while others are clergy or come from other backgrounds.

We use the word *viewer* to refer to the client, because it is the client, the viewer, who is doing the most important work in the session, that of viewing his or her own mental world. The facilitator assists in this process.

Within these pages, you may at times see the words *practitioner, therapist,* and *facilitator* being used interchangeably, depending on the viewpoint of the speaker/writer. Likewise you will see *client* and *viewer* used interchangeably.

Metapsychology (properly called Applied Metapsychology), includes the specific technique called Traumatic Incident Reduction. TIR addresses traumatic experiences to relieve any traumatic stress the client is carrying from that experience, bringing about a full resolution of the trauma, and often insights as well. Metapsychology techniques are used to address issues a client finds difficult but wants to deal with. Sometimes these techniques are used to address just the immediate thing the client has his or her attention fixated upon, such as a recent traumatic event, relationship difficulties, or a painful emotion of unknown origin. Some practitioners have the opportunity and training to use more techniques and address everything the client brings in as an issue, in each part of life. The whole process of working through these issues to a satisfactory conclusion is called Life Stress Reduction.

All Metapsychology techniques including TIR are done in a person-centered context. This is not quite the form of person-centered work developed by Carl Rogers, which is undirected. Rather, Metapsychology uses clear direction in the form of structured techniques to empower a client to look at the aspects of life that need attention in that client's opinion.

The person-centered context is established and upheld in several ways throughout the work. A practitioner takes up only those areas a client is willing and interested in addressing, refrains from comment, interpretation or advice, and consults with the client to make sure a satisfactory resolution has been achieved before ending the session. The work of Alice Miller is a powerful argument for working with clients of all ages in a fundamentally person-centered way.

We can demonstrate with TIR and its related techniques that childhood trauma can be resolved in adulthood. One interesting point to consider is that, while such resolution is undoubtedly valuable and desirable, achieving it much sooner after the trauma or distressing event occurs may be a significant improvement, certainly from the trauma sufferer's point of view. Much more work and research will be needed to demonstrate the effectiveness of techniques for which there is much anecdotal evidence.

TIR and Metapsychology practitioners adhere to rules of practice, called the Rules of Facilitation that hold the boundaries for this work. They use special exercises called the Communication Exercises in their training, in order to strengthen their ability to be fully present and non-judgmental at all times and to keep the session work flowing smoothly and well.

Each technique is taken to a satisfying end point for the client of whatever age, and the session overall is taken to a good end point, rather than ending according to a pre-determined time limit. You will see in these chapters that most of our authors find that children tend to reach end points significantly faster than adults. You might surmise that this is due to a child being less able to face the world and its pain and strife than adults are (though most people who practice TIR with children would say that they face things very well indeed), or that children reach end points faster because they have less stored up trauma to deal with than adults do. Theories aside, the client's experience of being done with an issue rules the day. Success builds upon success from one session to the next, culminating in the client arriving at a state of satisfaction, having dealt with the issues that prompted a reach for help.

There are many theories about what can and cannot be done effectively with children in a therapeutic setting. In addition to those ideas, some therapists believe that preverbal memory cannot be addressed with TIR since TIR involves having the client recount the experience of going through a traumatic incident, each time through.

In fact, preverbal incidents resolve as readily as later incidents. We can understand this when we consider that the client goes through and re-experiences the incident silently each time and then tells what happened. Children, having a shorter time from which to draw incidents than adults have, tend to go into preverbal incidents rather sooner than adults do. As you will see, this does not present a problem.

The biggest factor in determining whether a child (or an adult) is able to make use of TIR is his or her ability to focus attention on the material being addressed. As with adults, the stronger a child client's distress, the easier it is usually to engage him or her in the work. The preliminary use of lighter techniques first goes a long way toward establishing a person's readiness for TIR. You will see a variety of approaches in the interviews and articles that follow. Once again, all of the children's names and other identifying information have been changed.

The proof of this method is in the results, well illustrated in the case stories presented in this book. We do not just see clients saying, "I feel better now," though they do say that, of course. We also see children's general mood and behaviors change for the better after TIR and related techniques. Observable changes for the better, out in the real world, are the rewards of this work.

It is our hope that by collecting the wisdom of leading TIR practitioners on the vital subject of working with children, we have created a useful resource for practitioners and an inspiration to consider TIR training for those who have not yet had the opportunity. (See Appendix B for information on training.)

—Marian Volkman

January 15th, 2007

Part I:
Tools and Techniques

1

The Head Picture: Engaging Children in Incident-Specific Trauma Treatment

By Anna Foley, Clinical Director, Moorside Trauma Service, England

Engaging children in trauma treatment is primarily about helping them to talk about trauma, its symptoms, and its effects. Communicating information about stress reactions and the concept of mental/emotional treatment in an age-appropriate manner is crucial in showing that one can contain the horrors of trauma, and that one can be someone who will be able to help. This chapter lays out a technique I call 'The Head Picture'. I have been using it for over 10 years with child and adult clients, and have taught it to diverse audiences. It has never failed in improving the 'take up' of information in the clinical setting, when children and families are in crisis.

Inspiration for 'The Head Picture'

Without doubt my initial inspiration for this technique was Linda Chapman of Art Therapy Institute of the Redwoods (California), followed by the work of Robert Pynoos and Bessel van der Kolk.

The previous two decades have seen increasing evidence of the neurobiology of trauma. This has prompted my questioning of every aspect of my practice with traumatized children. The evidence regarding effects on the brain has revealed that areas associated with speech are reduced in size and functioning in traumatized children. This finding suggested to me that I ought to include information beyond the verbal realm in my communications with traumatized children and their families. I found that using images as well as speech has helped to demystify scary symptoms more efficiently and effectively. The impaired functioning after trauma also made me consider how one goes about gaining informed consent[1] from children and families. Informed consent with children is often difficult to obtain, but using words alone makes it doubly difficult. The use of images to convey post-traumatic stress reactions and therapy has been invaluable in getting to the point where the client is understood and feels understood, in gaining a more informed

---

[1] See the discussion on p. 23

consent, and in providing ways to measure a child's progress during therapy.

According to the Gerbode (1995) model (See Chapter 14), the TIR method is, "...in fact primarily educational in its intent." This differs from the traditional medical model of treatment vs. disease[2].

Starting as you intend to go on: handling the first appointment

If you work to get across an understanding of the concepts of stress and therapy, and set up an environment based on sharing knowledge and feelings, then the child is implicitly involved throughout. Children respond well to concrete examples of stress and its effects. Having been out of control during the traumatic experience, they need to receive useful knowledge and models from us so that they can separate their post-trauma reaction from themselves as people. If children are left with post trauma symptoms, they blame themselves for their inability to recover. This idea affects their self-esteem, and if left unaddressed, becomes an entrenched core belief. Entrenched shame is emotionally crippling and prolongs both suffering and trauma treatment. For complex traumas, this psychoeducation becomes a substantial part of the child's experience.

From the very first meeting, I convey that I welcome more than one way for the child to communicate with me. Another interpretation of this psychoeducation is that children are provided with something tangible. The picture they draw acts as an 'internalized transitional object' (many children take their drawing away with them), which they can use to externalize their post trauma symptoms.

---

[2] See "Applied Metapsychology: Therapy or Personal Growth?"
http://www.tir.org/metapsy/therapy.htm

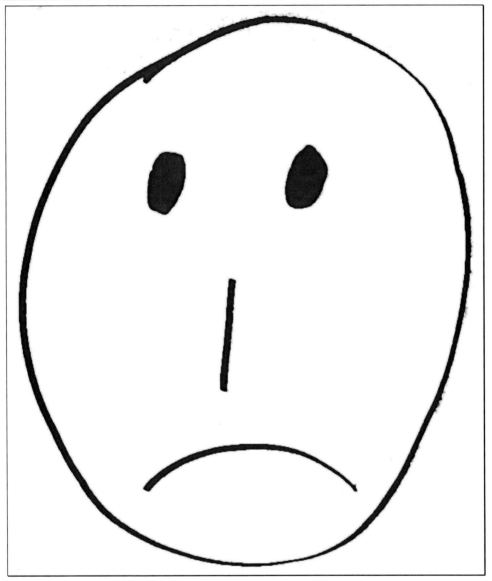

Fig. 1-1: Self-Image after an Incident (Head Picture)

'The Head Picture'

This is how I talk to children and families about trauma

T denotes me as therapist, **C** denotes child.

I might offer the child the choice of color as we pick out a felt-tip pen. I draw a simple picture of a sad face, sometimes just a line for the mouth if I am being cautious not to assume I know what the child is feeling.

T. "Let's say that this is you. I know it's not really anything like you; I'm not the best at drawing (*usually prompts a smile*). Let's say that this is you right after you were _____" (See Fig. 1-1.) *Here I will ascertain how the child describes or thinks of the traumatic experience: "stabbed," "shot," "beaten up," "attacked," etc. For complex trauma I generalize the stresses to be* "After all that's happened to you.")

The simple drawing and the fact it isn't perfect convey to the child that s/he does not have to be good at art to enter trauma treatment. I find children usually come with the pre-conceived idea that they have to do well, like at school. It is a good time also to tell the child that I am not a teacher.

Using the image gives them something to focus on while they are amid the anxiety of symptoms and the trepidation of the first appointment. Children and families visibly relax and are more receptive as soon as they see this 'funny' translation of stress into image.

The image sharing also allows a pacing which is fundamental in trauma treatment. In the introduction to treatment, I am attentive to the child's hyper-arousal, and watch carefully for raised heartbeat, sweaty palms, heightened startle response, etc. This gives me the opportunity to show the child and parent/caregivers how to calm themselves during post trauma arousal. It's crucial to show that treatment is paced so as to be tolerable to the child/client, and also to show that I expect these types of physiological changes to happen. Children then appear more able to actually talk about these symptoms during sessions.

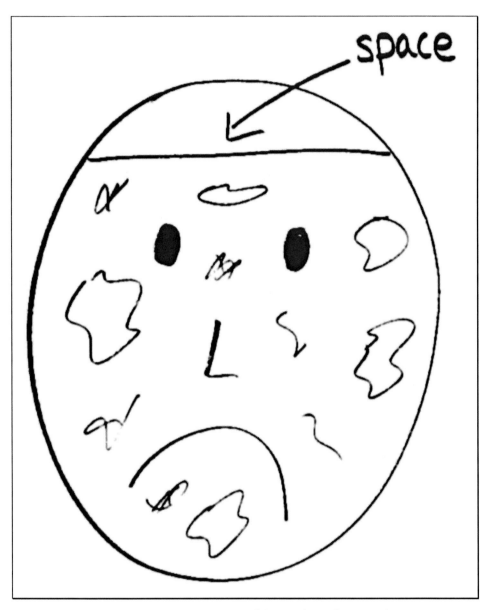

Fig. 1-2: Running Out of Space (Head Picture)

As a result of the psychoeducation beforehand, explaining to the child what we are going to do and what to expect, we are able to 'track sensation' during any exposure to the event(s) or other triggers that might arise.

T. "When someone is 'attacked' like you were, they find that they have lots and lots of thoughts, feelings and memories rushing round their mind, and body. Let's say these squiggly bits are all those different things (see Fig. 1-2). All different shapes and sizes, some small, some big, all feel different and some worse than others". *(Usually child and parent are nodding.)* "Is that how it is for you?"

I allow time to answer, and lots of information is shared at this point. This might have been the first time the family can begin to make some sense of what they have experienced and changes that they have noticed. I can also observe any stilted communications between family members, which the psychoeducation element of the therapy may help to overcome.

C. "Yeah, there's just all this stuff."

T. "When your head is busy trying to work out all of this stuff, it has only this little bit of space at the top, to think with or do things, that isn't full up of things already. So, when mum, dad or whoever asks you to do something like tidy your room, or do your homework, your little space becomes filled up and boom you 'explode'. Or you might get really cross..."

C. "That's what I do!" *(If the parents are there, they invariably say that the child wasn't like this before and he/she is now so hard to get on with, or that the simplest thing can trigger a rage.)*

T. "Well, you see, there's only this little bit of space to deal with every-day things, so when something else comes along, it sits in this little space; it fills it up, and Wham! Anger is usually the first reaction!" *(I go on to say that I'm not saying you should not do your homework or should break family rules, but that just now it's hard for you to follow them.)* "Mum, you might find that your head feels a little like this too, since you've had a great deal of stress to deal with also."

There is usually some discussion about how their family household is responding. It is pretty common from my experience that after a traumatic experience children appear extremely insecure, and don't want to leave their parents' side, or are withdrawing to their bedrooms much more than before.

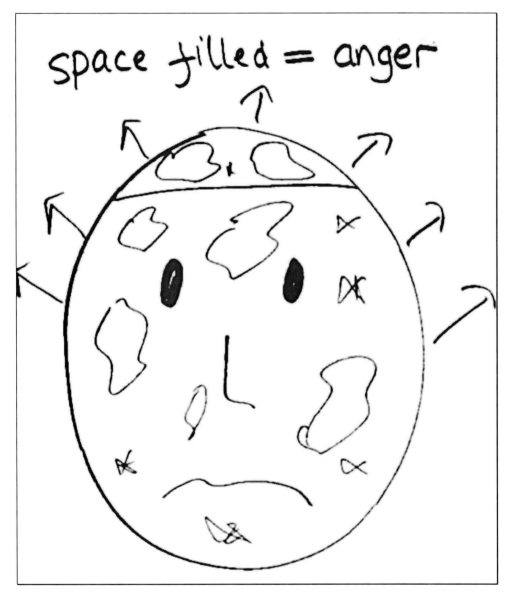

Fig. 1–3: Anger as a Result of Insufficient Space (Head Picture)

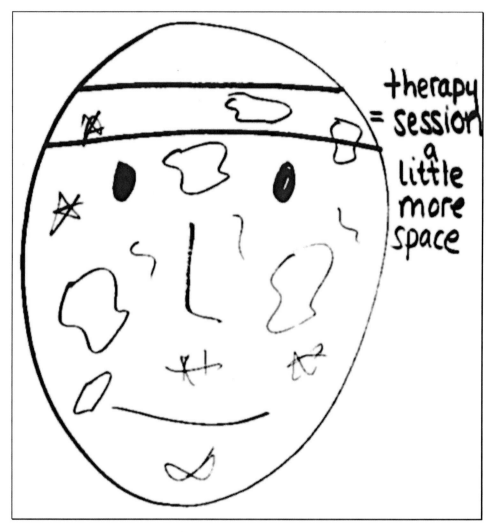

Fig. 1-4: After Initial Therapy (Head Picture)

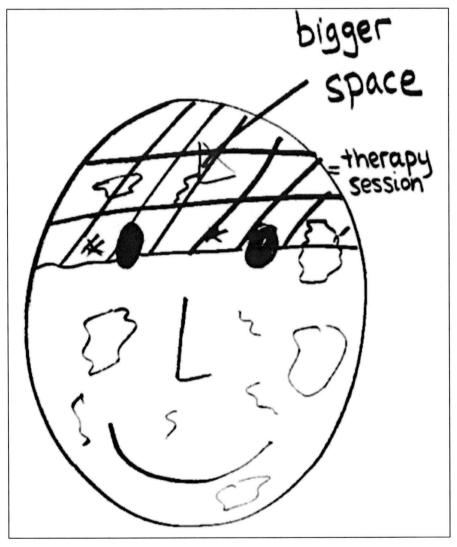

Fig. 1–5: After Initial Therapy Sessions are Complete

This is also an opportunity to explore the meaning of all the stuff they feel in their head and to include places in the body where there may be sensations or emotions. This is important so that we encapsulate the true impact of traumatic experience. Sometimes I might actually draw out a body outline.

T. "So this is a little like what it might feel like inside your head and your body. When someone like you comes to see someone like me, we do a little bit of looking at these different things. Sometime we might manage to do a couple of these things, sometimes only one or a bit of one. Sometimes by looking at one thing, another thing seems to disappear by accident."

T. "As time goes by, and you come here a few times, we will work together to make this space get bigger and bigger, and then you'll notice that everyday things get a bit easier; you'll have more and more space to do all your everyday things."

Most times children volunteer what the squiggles actually represent for them. It's useful also to put the trauma in relation to other stresses in their life. This usually includes other traumatic events, school issues, issues with parents, friends, etc.

T. "What we're aiming for when we do this work is to get to a time when you have lots of space to deal with your everyday things, and the terrible thing that has happened to you doesn't take up all the space in your head. It becomes a memory that doesn't hurt or frighten you like it does now. We can flip the 'Head Picture' over so that the big space is for you, and the little space is for the memories." (See Fig. 1-6)

Summary

If a child is consumed with anxiety around mummy leaving, worries about dying, nightmares, flashbulb or flashback memories, etc., then the child is unable to process fully what you are telling him or her. The therapist must demonstrate for the child that the therapeutic space is contained, that the therapist knows something about what the child is going through, and she or he is providing a way through the horror that doesn't necessarily need words. The therapist is providing a general tool to ascertain a unique trauma reaction. It also gives the family as a whole something to focus on and gives a tangible way of discussing stress together, whilst I'm not there to support that discussion.

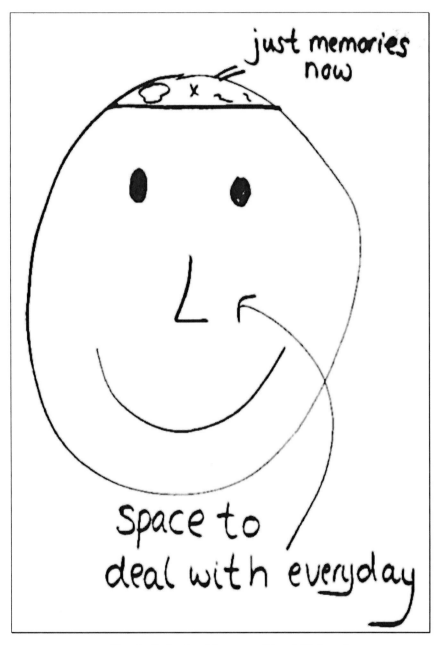

Fig. 1-6: Just a Memory (Head Picture)

The Head Picture as a measuring tool for children

The head picture also provides a way for children to reflect on their therapeutic goals. It gives the child and me a measuring tool, which can change over time. Shapes and sizes of things change, may become fewer, or even become more for a time, if there are other stressors in the child's life during treatment. Externalizing them to image form seems to produce a sense of management, mastery of expressed emotions, and encourages more calm.

A Child will often say...

C. "Do you remember 'The Head Picture' you showed me?"

T. "Yes, I remember."

C. "It looks more like this now." The child will invariably grab some paper and replicate the image and show that there is less 'stuff' in there.

I always double check this, and ask:

T. "Well OK great, we know it's not empty so what's in there now?" I am just checking out for anything left, and also conveying how ordinarily we have things that we think about or that trouble us, but that these everyday things are different from trauma.

A teenager I was working with after numerous gang attacks including beatings said at the end of his treatment, "My Dad still won't buy me a motorbike." I replied, "Crumbs! I might be an OK therapist, but I'm not *that* good. I'm afraid that you and your dad will have to sort that one out." He laughed, saying, "That's a shame. It was worth a try..."

To close the sessions I might offer the pen pot for the child to choose one, and ask him or her to put the trauma in the picture. It's usually the tiniest mark or shape and this gives me the opportunity to say "It's a memory now." (See Fig. 1-6)

Body Outline Images

Fig. 1-7 (on the following page) is the self-portrait made by a 13-year-old girl referred for TIR after being attacked by a gang of girls her own age, and having her tooth broken. This image imparts to the viewer that more has happened to this girl. Feelings in differing parts of her body are signified by red blobs, and the lines and 'belt' around her waist. It transpired that she had been raped many years before whilst in the care of the extended family, which was disclosed through images during and after running through TIR in image form.

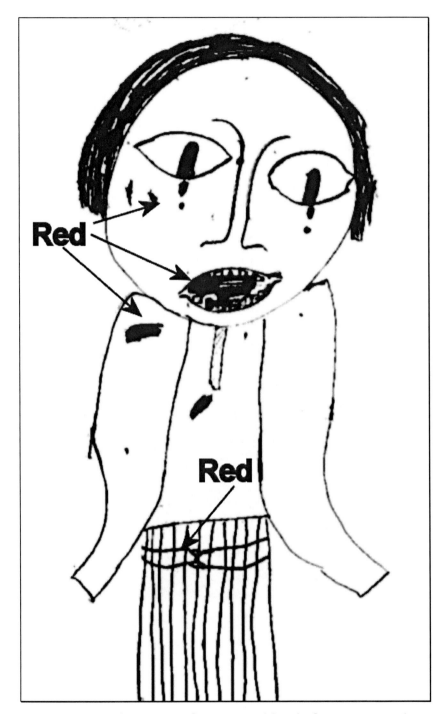

Fig. 1-7: Self-portrait of 13-year-old girl after gang attack

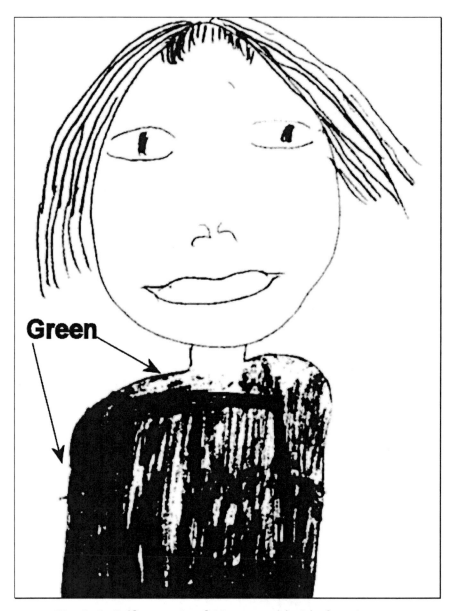

Fig. 1-8: Self-portrait of 13-year-old girl after therapy

Fig. 1-8 is a self-portrait that was produced after the initial incident was desensitized and older incidents were found and worked through in the same way.

Some examples of common symptoms that often arise amongst the scribbles, big and small

How would we discuss the symptoms with words alone?

- Intrusive re-experiencing: Images flashing in mind ("flashbulb memories", or flashbacks).

- Autonomic hyper-arousal: Increased heart rate, sweating.

- Sleep disturbances: Unable to fall asleep, or nightmares.

- Increased aggression: Angry more often, especially towards family.

- Separation anxiety: Clingy to mum or other family member.

- Avoidance of reminders of event: Children may want to stay in bedroom.

- Foreshortened future: Lost "shield of invincibility".

- Guilt: If child or family thinks they have done something wrong to cause the event.

- Revenge fantasies: These are common immediately after event, and can be scary to children, showing they are also capable of horrors towards others, at least in their minds.

- Why Me? "What is it about me that this was done to me?"

- What If? "What if he'd had a gun or a knife?" Children finish off their traumas in their mind's eye.

- If Only: "If only I'd gone home the way I should have gone," "If only I'd left with my friend." Child tries to make sense of why this happened.

- Traumatized family: All family members are affected even if only one member was directly involved. Children often experience a massive shift in the way the family works together, which further compounds their suffering. This is particularly the case in instances of rape and/or sexual abuse.

References

Andrews, B., et. al. (2000).'Predicting PTSD symptoms in victims of violent crime: the role of shame, anger, and childhood abuse. *Journal of Abnormal Psychology.* 109, 69-73.

Arguile, R., (1992) 'Art therapy with children and adolescents' in *Art therapy, a handbook* ed. by Waller D. & Gilroy A. Open University Press.

Betenksy, M. G., (1995).*What do you see? Phenomenology of therapeutic art expression* Jessica Kingsley Publishers (JKP).

Bisbey S & Bisbey L B. (1998). *Brief therapy for post traumatic stress disorder, Traumatic Incident Reduction and Related Technique.* Wiley

Bledkin, K. (1994). Post traumatic stress disorder once removed: a case report. *British Journal of Medical Psychology.* 67, 125-129.

Davidson, L. M. & Baum, A. (1994). Psychophysiological Aspects of Chronic Stress Following Trauma. In: Ursano, R. J., McCaughey, B. G., & Fullerton, C. S. (Eds.) *Individual and Community Responses to Trauma and Disaster: The Structure of Human Chaos.* Great Britain: Cambridge University Press, 1994.

Dyregrov A. et al (2000). Trauma exposure and psychological reactions to genocide among Rwandan children. *Journal of traumatic stress .* 13, 3-21.

Eth S. & Pynoos R.S. (1985). *Post traumatic stress disorder in children.* Arlington, VA: American Psychiatric Press

Eth S. & Pynoos R. S. (1994). Children who witness the homicide of a parent. *Psychiatry.* 57, 287-304.

Furnam E. (1986) When is the death of a parent traumatic? *The Psychoanalytical Study of the Child.* 41, 191-207.

Gelderm M. et. al. (1994). Classification of reactions to stressful experiences' in *Concise Oxford Textbook of Psychiatry, 4th Ed.* UK: Oxford University Press.

Gil E. (1991) *The healing power of play, working with abused children.* UK: The Guilford Press.

Heineman T V. (1998). *The abused child: Psychodynamic understanding and treatment.* UK: The Guilford Press

Herman J L. (1992). *Trauma and recovery: from domestic violence to political terror.* HarperCollins Publishers

Jung C G. (1964). *Man and his symbols.* Picador.

Kennedy H. (1986). Trauma in childhood. *Psychoanalytical study of the child.* 41, 209-219.

Kinchin D. (1994). *Post traumatic stress disorder.* New York: Harper-Collins Publishers.

Laor et al. (1998). The function of image control in the psychophysiology of post traumatic stress disorder. *Journal of Traumatic Stress.* 11:4, 679-696.

McCaughey, Hoffman, & Llewellyn (1994). The human experience of earthquakes in *Trauma and disaster* Cambridge University Press.

Mullarky K. & Pfeffer C. (1992). Psychiatric treatment of a child suicide survivor. *Crisis,* 13:2, 70-5.

Schavarien J. (1992). *The revealing image: analytical art psychotherapy in theory and practice.* Routledge.

Schavarien J. (1999). Art within analysis: scapegoat, transference and transformation. *Journal of analytic psychology.* 44, 479-510.

Silva R. et. al. (2000). Stress and vulnerability to post traumatic stress disorder in children and adolescents. *American Journal of Psychiatry.* 157, 1229-1235

Terr L C. (1991). Childhood Traumas: An outline and overview' *American Journal of Psychiatry.* 148:1, 10-19.

Van der Kolk, McFarlane & Weisaeth (1996). *Traumatic stress: the effects of overwhelming experience on mind, body and society.* The Guilford Press

Van der Kolk, B. (2005) Developmental Trauma Disorder. *American Psychiatric Annals.* 401-08

Vasarhelyi V. (1990.) Illness behaviour in children in *Working with children in Art Therapy* ed. by Case C. & Dalley T. Routledge.

Weine et al. (1997) Childhood trauma histories in adolescent inpatients. *Journal of Traumatic Stress.* 10:22, 291-298.

Weisbeski et al. 1989 'Urban Trauma: A recurrent disease' *Journal of trauma.* 29, 940-947.

Yule W. & Williams R. (1992) The management of trauma following disasters in *Child and Adolescent Therapy: a handbook* ed. by Lane D. & Miller A. Open University Press

2

TIR and Child Survivors
of Domestic Violence

A Conversation with Renee Carmody
as Interviewed by Marian K. Volkman

Marian: Tell us a little about your educational background before you became a clinician at VSC Miami.

Renee: I received a BA in Psychology from Florida International University and a Masters in Clinical Social Work from Barry University. I commuted 2 hours from Naples to Miami for my classes and internships, and the total miles I drove to receive my education were greater than the distance from the Earth to the Moon! The dedication I had toward my education was motivated only by my desire to work with children. That's all I knew... and I don't think I had a plan beyond that.

Marian: Tell us about your current position and what drew you to this field.

Renee: For the past six years, I've been working for Teresa Descilo and Shirley Hawkesworth at Victim Services Center (VSC) in Miami. During this time, I was promoted to Head Clinician and Training Director. Working at VSC has proved to be one of life's most precious gifts, but I don't think I chose the field... I think it chose me.

The day I was supposed to meet with my field advisor to determine my first placement, he was absent. Instead, there was a young doctoral student I think, who was filling in for him. I'll never forget what this guy said to me after our interview. He suggested that I would love to work at VSC because of my "healthy disrespect for distance." At the time, I didn't know what he meant by that, but now I get it! I have learned, through VSC that the greatest gift we can give to anyone is our presence.

I remember being totally fascinated by the information Teresa presented in the TIR workshop[1]. I also remember thinking, "How can this be?" It all sounded so simple: Let people tell you their story over and over, and they're going to be OK. I couldn't help but wonder why everyone wasn't using this technique?

---

[1] See Appendix C for information on training to become a TIR facilitator.

But what I loved most about the whole workshop was the "no inter-pretation, no analysis, and no judgment." Adapting this perspective and trying to live by it has improved every relationship I have in my life. And with practice I've been able to learn that no one was really looking for a hero, they just wanted someone to listen.

Marian: You have kids coming in to see you who are in a really bad situation. For example, their family could be breaking up, there may be domestic violence, and everything is in upheaval. How do you get them ready to be in session and concentrate to do the work?

Renee: Actually, the way we have the kids set up right now is that we see them on Saturdays. We have a children's group that goes from 1 pm to 4 pm. During those three hours, the first hour used to be arts & crafts, but we now do work based on *Awakening the Heroes within: Twelve Archetypes to Help Us Find Ourselves and Transform Our World* by Carol Pearson (1991). In her model, everyone has heroes inside them: Innocent, Orphan, Warrior, Caregiver, Seeker, Destroyer, Lover, Creator, Ruler, Magician, Sage, and the Fool. We give the kids two he-roes a week and they think of a time that they were one of these (e.g. the Caregiver) and draw a picture of it. For kids' drawings, we use the "What are you saying?" and "What are you thinking?" bubbles. This works well because they don't understand to protect themselves or change what they are saying or thinking in front of you. They *really* tell you what they are thinking.

The second hour is dance and the third hour is yoga. All kids go through the groups, but if they don't want to, we can set up individual sessions. However, most of them love the group setting. Within those three hours, we pull the kids in for individual counseling sessions. That way we can see twice as many with our afternoon activity structure as we could in conventional counseling. As you know, normally when you see a kid for 60 minutes' time; 30 minutes is hard work for them and 30 minutes is fun time for them. With the groups, we pull them out for the 30 minutes of hard work and then they go back for the fun. There-fore we can see twice as many for the real work of the one-on-one sessions.

Marian: That seems like a good idea.

Renee: Yes. We also tell them during admission exactly what we ex-pect from them. There isn't anybody who comes into the agency that doesn't understand what the agency does. The focus is going to be talk-ing about all the terrible things they've seen or had done to them.

Marian: OK. Do they seem to be accepting of this help?

Renee: Well, one of the important things in our protocol is what we tell them about it. They will come into admissions and they'll be crying and really unhappy about being there and don't understand why they're there. I give them the systems theory (what social workers believe): that your problem doesn't have anything to do with you, it's because of all the bad things you've seen. As soon as we can get them to understand that we don't believe that there's anything wrong with them, it really eases them up. I have no doubt the parent has often told them that, "You've got a problem and you're going to have to do something about it".

The children are usually unsure of the situation: I always ask, "Do you know why you are here?" and invariably at least 90% say they don't know. I ask, "Do you know what counseling is?" and they say that they don't know. Personally, I can remember when I was a child and Health and Human Services got involved in our lives. I asked my mother why we had to go to that place and she said "Because they think you're nuts!"

Marian: Very helpful, right?

Renee: I was very cautious the whole time I was there to not say anything to make me sound like I was nuts. So I doubt that the experience of children coming to our center is much different, because they are devastated that they have to be there.

Marian: What are the limits of confidentiality and children with regards to informed consent?

Renee: Immediately following introducing yourself to the child, it is important that you inform the child of the limits of confidentiality. They need to understand what can be kept secret and what cannot be kept a secret. Make sure you have the child's full attention and that she or he understands what you have said. Explain that if s/he tells you any of these things, then you will have no choice except to report it and make sure it doesn't continue to happen.

Often times, you will be the first counselor with whom the child has ever spoken. Failure on your part to ensure the child understands the limits of confidentiality may later be viewed as a sense of betrayal, especially if you are placed in the situation of having to report any suspected or real abuse by a family member or friend.

It is also important to include the parent (we usually only work with one parent in domestic violence situations) in this part of the process, to ensure that they understand your obligation to report as well as your perceived obligation to not disclose any other confidential issues the child may present. We inform the parent that the laws in our state (Florida) do not protect the confidentiality of a child's session from the parent. In order to gain the most from this intervention, ask the parent (in front of the child) if s/he will be able and willing to respect the privacy of the sessions. If the parent agrees, then the child will hold her (or him) to that agreement. That empowers the child to share all of his or her experiences with you.

Marian: How do you explain the nuts and bolts of session work to the children?

Renee: The method you use to explain the TIR process should be age appropriate. This simply means that you do not use any terminology or concepts that are above the child's level of understanding. It seems, regardless of age, that everyone understands the concept, "It's like watching a videotape, rewinding it, and then watching it again." Tell child clients that they are going to be telling you the story "over and over and over and over and over" until it stops hurting. Make sure children understand the importance of repetition and prepare them to feel everything they felt during the traumatic experience. The more children understand what to expect, the more they will engage in the process. Following is an example of the dialogue that could be presented as a means to explain TIR:

> "I've already told you, you are here because of all the bad things that have happened to you. What we're going to do together is make a list of those bad things and then work on them one at a time. After we make the list, you get to pick which you want to work on first. Then, I'm going to ask you to make a movie in your head of what happened in that one.
>
> You see, our brains can't tell the difference between imagination and reality. So, if you close your eyes, you're sometimes going to feel like it's really happening again, but it's not. You'll be here in the office with me, and this is a safe place. And the only thing I'm here to do is help guide you through your story and just listen. I'm not going to tell you what I think you should think, or what I think really happened, I'm not you. I just need you to watch the movie and tell me what happened.
>
> Then I'm going to ask you to watch again and tell me what happened, and you're going to keep doing this over and over and over, until you can watch the whole thing and it

doesn't bother you anymore. The thing I also need you to remember is that if you got a stomach ache when the incident happened, then you'll probably get a stomach ache again, but it won't last long. Just plan on it."

When working with adolescents, their normal response seems to be, "It's the same thing." Explain to them up front that the story details may not change, but that's not what you're looking for. Tell them that it's OK if they keep telling you the same thing over and over; you're not going to get bored. You just want to make sure they include all the details every time they tell the story, and that's all that is important.

Marian: I've found even with adults that the instruction, "close your eyes" can be a problem. Since TIR is a non-hypnotic technique, there is no strict reason for eyes to be closed. Many of us just tell new clients (of whatever age) when we are explaining what we're going to do, that they *may* close their eyes when going through the incident, *if they wish.* I'm guessing that children may have even more problems with this instruction.

Renee: Yes, when working with a child, even mentioning that he or she will have to close their eyes during the process seems to create an immediate sense of heightened anxiety and the process itself becomes as scary as the incident.

Maybe this is due to the child's lack of well-developed coping skills to distance themselves from the reality and emotions connected with the incident, but it is clear they have no 'brakes' in place to ease them into the emotions and sensations connected with the incident. For some children, the simple task of closing their eyes slams them into the moment and it becomes too much, too fast. I have learned that it's OK if the child doesn't want to close his/her eyes. It works better if they are not looking at you. Otherwise, they will pace their story with the speed of your ability to write everything down and the process loses its intended focus. So for example you might suggest that they look at a (blank) wall while re-experiencing the incident.

Marian: Are there other techniques you use to improve their ability to focus without becoming overwhelmed?

Renee: Allowing children to keep their eyes open and have them engage in some right-brain activity during the process seems to create a slowing device for the child while still accessing the memories and emotions of the traumatic incident. Smaller children enjoy playing with the doll house or setting up the farm or circus animals. Older children work the process very well while creating beadwork. If an adolescent chose to do nothing, I gave them silly putty to play with during the process. The twisting and pulling on the silly putty as they run through the incident seems to eliminate their irritability with the process itself and their focus remains on the incident.

What has been fascinating to observe as children reach the same state of mind that they were in at the time of the incident is their willingness to stop what they're doing, squeeze their eyes shut, hunch their shoulders, and go through the incident holding that posture really tightly as they repeat the process a of couple times. Then, without prompting, they open their eyes and resume playing as they continue with another repetition until they reach an end point. Following is an example of how the process develops, but the actions that took place have been duplicated with both girls and boys and at various ages.

Example: An 8-year-old girl was referred to the agency after having been molested by a family friend. While in the limousine of a funeral procession, the child was placed on the lap of the family friend. During the ride between the funeral parlor and cemetery the man reached under her dress and fondled her. As the child described all that was happening, she methodically played with the doll house during the first four times through. On the fifth time through, she stopped what she was doing, closed her eyes tightly, hunched her shoulders and continued through to the end, and did the same the next time through, holding this position. On the seventh time through, she opened her eyes, resumed play and went through the incident five more times. After the tenth time through, she began to giggle and stated, "It doesn't bother me anymore," and the session was over.

Marian: Thanks for that example. I understand that you work with wrong indications with these children.

Definitions

Indication: A deliberate assertion about something related to a person's case, personality, situation or condition.

Wrong Indication: **(WI)** An evaluative and generally invalidative statement that violates the recipient's self-concept and perception of what is true.

(The subject of wrong indications is taught on the second-level TIR Workshops.)

Renee: In the main, we do TIR on the incident where that belief was formed. Now they can see for themselves that it's not true. If I were to tell them myself it wasn't true, I would just be another adult telling them "That's not true," but with TIR, they can figure this out for themselves, and it gives them their power back.

Marian: What kind of wrong indications do these kids receive from people around them?

Renee: Often with recovering addicts, as an example, a girl is placed in the custody of her grandmother. I don't understand it, but the grandmother then says to her quite commonly, "You're gonna grow up to be a whore like your mother." That's a wrong indication and devastating to the kids. I can't tell you how many times I've helped them work through that one. Obviously the lack of parenting skills shows, but the adult is trying to scare the kids away from that behavior. In the meantime, it's destroying the kid.

Marian: It might be an effort to help but it's certainly not the best way.

Renee: No, it's not working! Additionally, lots of wrong indications occur without ever being said. A primary cause of this is that children are not told the whole story of an event age-appropriately. So when things happen, they end up using their own imagination and often create their own wrong indications. Combine that with a child's own natural ego-centric thinking at that age and they make up that *everything* is their fault.

Marian: How should a traumatic event be explained to a child?

Renee: Age-appropriately, but the *whole* story. One of my most interesting cases was with a mother and a child. I love working with a parent and a child because I can see the same incident from each of their perspectives, which is so cool. In this particular incident, the child was in a boot camp. There are different levels of boot camps in Florida and this one was a "no touch" facility, but they were beating the kids anyway. As a result of everything that happened, that camp eventually closed. This boy was sixteen years old, a juvenile delinquent, a high school dropout, and using drugs. His mother got him out of the camp and brought him to the agency. He came to the session (after intake) and I asked him, "What would you like to work on first?"

He says, "Well, my sister died."

I'm thinking, "I hadn't heard anything about this!" but I said instead "OK. How old were you when your sister died?"

"Two years old."

"OK, well then let's do that," I said.

Because bad memories are held in bits and pieces and over the course of time he had never been told anything about his sister's death, he had formed the belief (or given himself a wrong indication) that it was his fault that his sister had died. He had a memory of when he was two years old at that time; that alone was fascinating to me. The bits and pieces that he did remember, he remembered very well. The first time through in TIR he said that he was lying on the floor and his baby sister, who was six months old, was lying on his belly and sucking on his finger. He remembered that the baby had convulsions, went to the hospital, and died.

Right after that that he was sent to across the country to live with his grandparents and nobody ever talked to him about it. To further reinforce this belief that he was at fault, at age six he and his mother were sitting on the couch looking at the photo album. He said to his mother, "Who is that?" and she said "That's your sister" and she left the room crying. That only reinforced his belief that he'd done something wrong.

As we did TIR over several iterations, things started changing. Yes, he was in the living room, but the baby was not on his chest; instead, she was in a crib and he was watching TV. Then he remembered that his mother went to the phone and called the father home from work. All four of them then went to the hospital. Whether he remembered it during the original incident or not, he at some point heard that the baby had a pinhole in her heart and was going to need lots of surgery. That's why he was sent to live with the grandparents while his mother and father basically lived at the hospital, during the surgeries with the baby. The next time he remembered seeing his mother, everyone was in black, and everyone was crying. After many more iterations of the story changing from his dreams and imaginations to reality, he realized that it wasn't his fault. What a great relief it was for him! Some of the things that you see on people's faces make you think, "My whole life has been worth it just to see the relief on this poor child's face!"

Later I saw the mother and I had previously told her, "We don't see a child unless the parent comes in. No exceptions." If the parent says, "I'm fine," I explain to them about secondary traumatization. In this case, I'd say, "Let's go through the incident on your son's beating. Eventually, the mother came in for her session and I said, "Let's go to work on that incident of your son's beating." She said, "I'd rather work on when my daughter died." So they were both stuck there! Of course I said, "OK."

During the original intake, she had said repeatedly about her son: "He's different, he's different." I had asked her before this, "When do you think your son changed?" She said, "When he was about age two." I thought to myself, "Wow, that was his age when his sister died." We proceed to do TIR addressing the incident of the daughter dying, from her perspective. In going through the incident, when she got the part where they went to the grandparents' after the daughter died, she recognized for the first time: "I had no idea where my son was. I don't remember holding him. I don't remember who was taking care of him." She had just been lost in her own grief and didn't recognize how the incident affected her son. So it was from that long absence and the lack of telling the child age-appropriately what happened that their lives changed for the next fourteen years. Now they're both doing great and communicating. It's almost like they were on such different levels before doing TIR that they couldn't communicate before completing the incident.

There is another similar mother-and-son case where both of them were much older. This mother said: "He changed when he was six or seven. I don't think he was ever able to develop empathy; he just seemed so cold." When I did TIR with her son, it turned out that when he was age six or seven, his dog had died and his mother wasn't there. Meanwhile, I found out from his mother that at that date she had been recently divorced, going back to college, and studying for exams when the dog died. So again, it's just from a lack of communication, or sometimes *any* communication, or from bad communication that kids pick up these wrong indications.

Marian: It sounds as though you get into TIR pretty quickly with the children you see.

Renee: Very quickly. Kids are for the most part very eager to do it.

Marian: What age range do you see for TIR?

Renee: I try not to do TIR with anyone under age 5. They have to be able to understand that they're going to have to repeat the story over and over; they have to understand that they might get a bellyache or have other uncomfortable feelings. If they're not at that level of development, then we can't do it. What we do provide for kids who are not at that age-appropriate level is to have them draw the experience and then they tell me about it. And then they tell me about it again until it gets lighter for them. For those under age 5, creating the movie in their mind and repeating it over and over and over can be a problem. I think there was only one 4-year-old whom I actually tried it with. 5-year-olds can potentially understand TIR, but from age six on, they really get it.

Marian: Do you see differences in the way children vs. adults respond to TIR?

Renee: Yes, I'd say the average amount of time for TIR with children (off the top of my head) is between 20 and 30 minutes. Children have a much better ability to focus on the incident. There hasn't been that stage of analyzing and interpreting that adults do. You just keep redirecting them back. They see the incident; they tell you what happened; they see the incident again and tell you what happened, etc.

Marian: So they're not busy analyzing it and figuring out what it all means?

Renee: Yes, that's right.

Marian: That's a really interesting observation, because when I talk to some therapists about this, they theorize that children would not be as able to do TIR as well as adults.

Renee: That theory is incorrect; they can do it so well! It doesn't matter what the incident is either. A lot of our kids are witnesses or victims of domestic violence. We've had homicide survivors who have witnessed one of their parents being killed. We get lots of kids who are the children of recovering addicts and the stories that they live through are horrendous. They've witnessed their mother being beaten with brass knuckles or a machete, you name it.

Marian: What kind of outcomes do you get?

Renee: I anticipated that question and looked up some end points[2] from past TIR sessions. The first case is of a 16-year-old boy whose mother had died during his birth. His father, who was later diagnosed as a schizophrenic, raised him alone. We did TIR on an incident where, as a 7-year-old boy, he had to kneel on the stones of the driveway on his bare knees for eight hours as part of his discipline. When he got done reviewing this incident he said, "I don't feel anything, it feels good."

Marian: Did you note how long that case took?

---

[2] The *end point* is the specific point at which TIR and related techniques are finished, recognizable because the client feels complete and satisfied with that piece of work; the client looks brighter and possibly has realizations or other perceptual or cognitive shifts; and (most importantly) the client's awareness comes fully into the present.

Renee: He was pretty average for his age, so he was between 30 and 40 minutes for a complete TIR session.

Case #2 was a 16-year-old boy from a lockdown facility as a runaway. He kept saying "My dog died" over and over, and he was crying. I thought to myself, "What a sensitive kid." So we went and did TIR on the incident. His dog was his best friend, but I didn't know that at the time. His "friend" had been electrocuted on the way to school. His end point was, "Let it be; it happened. You can't change the force of nature."

Case #3, was another 16-year-old boy in a stabbing incident, not gang-related or anything. My client and his sister were walking down a street and a guy walking by said something to the girl. This resulted in an argument. The guy beat him up and stabbed the sister. My client reacted by delinquent-like behavior and was transferred to an alternative school. There was no place we could meet in the school that wouldn't be interrupted by a bell. So we actually went out in my truck, with permission from the school, and did TIR in there, parked on the baseball field. His end point was "It seems lighter 'cause I don't think about it now. I'm feeling like I'm alright, Miss." Then he started laughing, that laughing kind of relief. Then he said "I'm happy again, Miss. Is that what you do for people, just listen and let them go over and over it?" He started laughing again and said, "It's off my chest now, Miss."

Case #4, was an 8-year-old girl who said, "It doesn't hurt no more" as the end point.

Case #5, was a 15-year-old girl who had been gang-raped. By the time she got done at the end of the session, her end point was, "It's not my fault. I remembered so many things I totally forgot."

Marian: It's great to hear your stories! The youngest client I've ever had for TIR was six years old and I considered that he was a remarkable child. Now after hearing this, I'm revising my opinion...

Renee: If they're capable of understanding it, then they're going to keep telling you the movie over and over and staying engaged until the end point. Recently, there was the case of a 4-year-old girl who had witnessed a homicide. Her cousin had been shot in front of her and her mother was shot in the face (but didn't die). I couldn't do TIR with her of course, because of her age. However, one of the greatest things is that I get to teach the parents some key points in the group session "The Effects of Domestic Violence on Children." I teach them the Communication Exercises (See Glossary), and tell them that children will only tell you as much as they think you can handle. I met with the father of this little girl and her soon-to-be stepmother. I said, "I can't do

TIR with her, but the best I can do for her is to prepare you to hear her story. You guys have got to practice this so that whenever she wants to talk about it, she can."

You would never have guessed that this girl had been through everything that she had. She had witnessed horrendous domestic violence between her mother and her mother's boyfriend. The father said that during the five-hour drive to take her home from the center, she was in the back car seat. Because it was dark, she couldn't see her father's face and his reaction, so she told him the entire story. The father told me, "Oh my God, I'm so glad I drove her back at night because I was crying. But I didn't say anything and she just told me everything that happened." She couldn't see his responses and that's why she didn't stop. I really think that was the healthiest and greatest thing that could have happened for them.

My work with her was through pictures and she had drawn a picture of this terrible person and her memory of what had happened. For example, I asked her to draw a picture of her family. She drew herself and her mommy on one side of the page. Because she loved to cut-and-paste, she cut it out and pasted as expected. She looked at me and said, "I'm going to put so-and-so on the other side of the paper." She drew him and a baby on his side. I said, "Well, I didn't know he had a baby?" She said "No, that's a pretend baby, but we'll give him one."

Then we talked about domestic violence and what was against the law and what wasn't (age-appropriately) and helped her understand why she was living with her daddy and not her mother, and how her mother needed to get help, and stuff like that. I was really trying to pave the way for her understanding. About two to three weeks later, we were in the room and she was doing her cut-and-paste and she said "Do you still have that picture of so-and-so?" I said, "Yeah." She said "I don't have bad dreams about him no more. He's in jail." I said "Oh, OK, great!" So I got her the picture and she drew a circle around him and bars and put him in jail. I really think she was done with it at that point. It's pretty cool.

Marian: What kind of measurements do you do in terms of pre- and post-testing?

Renee: When working with a child (before TIR), it seems our first interests automatically focus on gaining a better understanding of what the child is feeling. However, what we sometimes forget is that although the child may know where in their body they have had that sensation, they may not know *what* to call it. We go through the Emotions Chart based on Gerbode (1995) *[The Emotional Scale in Fig. 2-1 with illustra-tions. –Ed.]*, and give examples of each state: frustration, anger, happiness, excitement, surprise, nervousness. You ask the kid, "What are the emotions you have?" We give them examples so they clearly understand, and ask them where they feel it in their bodies so they really get it.

ELATION
ENTHUSIASM
CHEERFULNESS
CONSERVATISM
COMPLACENCY
CONTENTMENT
AMBIVALENCE
ANTAGONISM
ANGER
RESENTMENT
HIDDEN HOSTILITY
ANXIETY
FEAR
GRIEF
APATHY

Fig. 2–1: The Emotional Scale

Fig. 2-2 (see p. 32) shows an example of a mandala (from Buddhism, a circular representation of the person's world). The mandala is a great tool to help the child identify those feelings he or she has already experienced and to learn the word that is used to describe that feeling. We write down everything the child identifies, there is no right or wrong answer. Examples of feelings can include, but are not limited to: happy, sad, mad, angry, nervous, excited, and nothing. Being completely person-centered, we don't coach them on what a feeling is and we just allow them to use their own vocabulary. After completing the list, we instruct the child to pick the color that represents that feeling and fill in the circle next to its name. Following this task, we explain to the child we want them to pretend the big circle is them, and we'd like them to show how much of them is mad, how much of them feels 'nothing', and so on. Once the mandala is complete, it becomes a great tool to build the child's Charged Area List. Thus

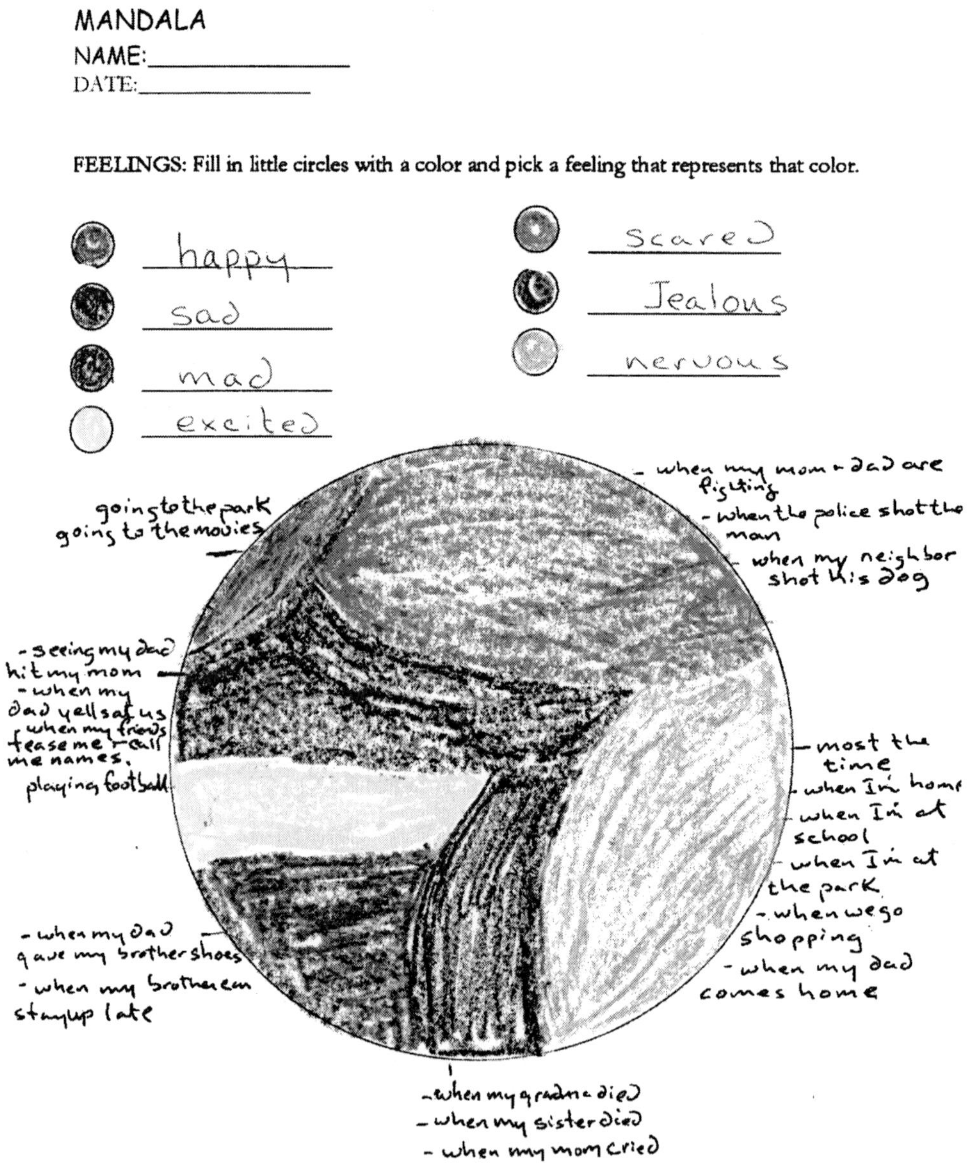

MANDALA

NAME:_____

DATE:_____

FEELINGS: Fill in little circles with a color and pick a feeling that represents that color.

◉ _happy_   ◉ _scared_

◉ _sad_   ◉ _Jealous_

◉ _mad_   ◉ _nervous_

○ _excited_

going to the park
going to the movies

- when my mom + dad are
  fighting
- when the police shot the
  man
- when my neighbor
  shot his dog

- seeing my dad
  hit my mom
- when my
  dad yells at us
- when my friends
  tease me + call
  me names.

  playing football

- most the
  time
- when I'm home
- when I'm at
  school
- when I'm at
  the park
- when we go
  shopping
- when my dad
  comes home

- when my dad
  gave my brother shoes
- when my brother can
  stay up late

- when my grandma died
- when my sister died
- when my mom cried

**Fig. 2-2: Mandala Diagrams Drawn by Child To
Illustrate Current Emotional State**

we can drive the session by asking them, "Tell me a time you were mad", "Tell me a time when you were happy", etc.

Many kids can graph it better than they can explain it. For example, they might be 75% scared and 25% nervous and they don't even have anything else on it.

We also use several other scales and for the pre-, mid-, and post-testing at VSC Miami:

- *Child Report of Post-traumatic Symptoms* (CROPS) (Greenwald and Rubin, 1999) – with a clinical cut-off of 19

- *The Depression Self-Rating Scale* (Birleson, 1981) – 13

- *Self-Concept Scale for Children* (Lipsitt, 1958)

- *Youth Coping Index* (McCubbin, Thompson, and Elver) – acceptable range -91.8 to 95.4

They're all generally Likert scales (a psychometric scale where the respondent must choose specific levels like "frequently", "always", "never" and so on). The scales generally talk about their ability to focus, how often they 'space out', how well can they concentrate...

Marian: Can you mention any particular outcome successes these scales have quantified?

Renee: There is a girl, aged eleven, who witnessed domestic violence between her stepfather and mother. Her case is still in progress as of this interview. Pre-tests showed lots of depression, low self-concept, and high on the PTSD scale. It turned out we only needed to do one TIR session on each of the two worst incidents she had seen. The first incident was when her mother was pregnant and the guy slammed the mother on the ground, broke everything in the house, and so on. We did another similar incident and then mid-tested her after about six hours total of session time. All of her PTSD symptoms were gone at that point as a result of TIR, but her self-concept score was off and her depression level was still high.

I said, "Help me understand what is going on here?" She said, "I'm fat and ugly." Now we have to discover when the first time she formed the belief that she was ugly. Of course, she's not ugly, she's a little chubby but she's eleven years old for goodness sake. I asked her, "When was the first time you formed that belief?" and then we worked on that. She said, "The adults are always saying that I'm not fat and I'm beautiful, but that's not what my friends say. My friends tease me." The next time I see her, I'm going to use TIR addressed to the incidents of her friends saying that and she's probably going to conclude that "They're stupid," or something like that. The tests really represent the incidents that support the negative beliefs, which I find very interesting. The children repair on the tests as effectively and successfully as adults when they've done their full sessions.

Kids don't have a lot "stuff", you know what I mean? You get three or four of the 'big bang' sessions and they are good to go. They don't have a lot of similar incidents to work on and it's all very short-term. A child can be done with Life Stress Reduction in five or six sessions and they are ready to go on with life.

Marian: Are there any other things you'd like to add?

Renee: We also use Future TIR with children as part of developing their Safety Plan. The reality of some of these kids is that they are going to have visitation with their father and this is the man they had witnessed nearly beat or choke their mother to death. Their fears are real so we help them develop a Safety Plan.

In one case, I took the girl outside and showed her how to read street signs (she was eight) and then made sure she memorized her mother's work number. She was three or four years old the last time she'd seen her father, but now she could take care of herself much better. This little girl's fear was that the father was going to kidnap them. He had been gone for a few years and then had received visitation rights from the court.

You have to educate the kids first on "Here's what we can do," then do Future TIR on the worst thing that could happen. She said, "The worst thing that's going to happen is daddy is going to come to school and take us." We had already talked about it: "You're going to say 'OK' and you're not going to argue with your father." You sort of build the story with them. While doing Future TIR she said, "My sister and I are in the back seat and I tell my daddy that I'm thirsty. He says, 'Well, wait until we get to California'. My sister is crying and crying. I tell her, 'Just say, OK.' We say, 'OK.'"

Another time though: "Now it's two or three weeks later and my daddy is standing at the window watching us at school and we can't tell anybody what's going on. Then one day, he decides he has to go to work. I'm in school, so I go up to the teacher and say, "My daddy kidnapped us and this is my mother's work number."'

They keep telling the story over and over again, making a movie of the worst thing that's going to happen and it makes it OK. It gives them a plan and they become very comfortable with the whole thing.

Marian: Thank you Renee, for your time and for a fascinating interview!

References

Gerbode, Frank A. (1995). *Beyond Psychology: An introduction to Metapsychology, 3rd Ed.* Menlo Park: IRM Press.

Pearson, Carol (1991). *Awakening the Heroes within: Twelve Archetypes to Help Us Find Ourselves and Transform Our World.* San Francisco: Harper.

Self concept scale for children [SC] (1958). Lipsitt LP. in Corcoran K & Fischer J (2000*). Measures for clinical practice: A sourcebook. 3rd Ed.* (2vols.) NY, Free Pr. V.1,Pg.617-618

Youth coping index [YCI] (1995). McCubbin HI; Thompson A; Elver K. IN: Corcoran K & Fischer J (2000). *Measures for clinical practice: A sourcebook. 3rd Ed.* (2 vols.) NY, Free Pr. V.1,Pg.628-631

TIR and Working with Children: Training Supplement

By Teresa Descilo, MSW

Victim Services Miami

[Note from the Editor: The following section is reproduced from the protocol document "TIR and Working with Children." Specifically, these are things besides TIR that are involved in working with children as clients: pre-/post testing Subjective Units of Distress (SUDs), basic techniques for children who are not ready for TIR, and the handling of misdeeds. We gratefully acknowledge Victims Services Miami for permission to reproduce it in this volume. To get the ideal results from these techniques, at least the first level of training, the TIR Workshop, Level One, is recommended.]

Obtaining the Subjective Units of Distress (SUDs)

WHEN YOU THINK ABOUT IT NOW... How bad is the feeling?

"On a scale of 0 to 10, 0 is no bad feeling, up to 10, the worst feeling. Circle a number to show how much bad feeling there is **right now**, when you think about the event."

---

0 - 1 - 2 - 3 - 4 - 5 - 6 - 7 - 8 - 9 - 10

(No bad feeling)... (Worst feeling)

Fig. 2–3: Subjective Units of Distress Scale (SUDS)

Due to the subjectivity of feelings, the scale in Fig. 2-3 is shown to clients so they might choose the number that identifies the severity of the emotions or lack of emotions still connected with the incident. However, when working with children, some may be too young to understand the concept behind the scale, but you still have to obtain some form of measurement indicating how distressing the incident is to the child prior to TIR, and how much those feelings have changed due to the process.

With smaller children, you can spread your arms apart and ask them, "How much does it bother you now?" They understand that concept and will join you in spreading their arms to indicate the level of anxiety the incident still holds. You continue to use this scale through the process itself.

Normally we ask an adult, "Does the incident seem lighter, heavier, or the same?" Small children will not understand what you mean, and sometimes adolescents don't understand what you mean either. You have to work with all children to determine their concept of a lot and a little. Adolescents seem to replace the words "lighter" and "heavier" with "It's easier", or "It's harder."

Example: There was a case with a 5-year-old boy who had been traumatized when he learned that his 10-year-old sister had been molested by his father. Unfortunately, when his mother told him this story, she included all of the graphic details and the visualization the child created went beyond his ability to process the information. This resulted in trauma for him.

Prior to TIR, he indicated that his upset was as big as his arms could spread themselves away from each other. As the TIR session continued, he stopped using his arms and eventually began to indicate his degree of upset using a distance between his index finger and thumb, continuously showing me the gap that existed between his finger and thumb until there was only a quarter inch space... and then the space was gone after what he determined to be his last repetition. After he finished, he looked at me and asked, "Is it OK if I don't like my father anymore?" I replied, "You can handle it anyway you want". And then he replied, "I don't think I want him as my father anymore, and I got a good father now." The session was over.

Children and False Beliefs

Once the mandala is complete and the child has a better understanding of the emotions he or she has experienced, you can begin to take the history. As you take the child's history, with any child who is manifesting anger, rage, suicidal ideation, or depression, please check for and handle false beliefs, wrong interpretations and indications. Children are victimized in this way all the time: "You're stupid," "You'll never amount to anything," "You're no good," "You make me unhappy," etc. In the case of suicidal thoughts or attempts, major rages or sudden depression, ask the child to think about the time just before feeling that way and ask if any one gave him/her a false belief or wrong indication and handle each one with the appropriate techniques.

Children also employ a type of magical thinking that seems to give them super powers. They believe that with these powers, they could have stopped the bullet that killed their brother, or prevented their mother from going out the front door where she was killed. Explore how they would have achieved this. Do a role play and have them recreate the scene and verbalize each step they would have taken. A child's thinking is pretty concrete and they will be more successful at solving problems if they can be clearly tied to physical reality.

Most children are anxious and ready to perform TIR. However, please use the following techniques if the child is resistant to the counseling itself.

Definitions

Unblocking: A procedure in which a number of mental blocks on a certain issue are addressed repetitively until charge has been reduced on that subject. (See p. 176 for an overview)

Person and Family Action Drawings

This is another type of diagnostic tool that can be used to measure self-image and family dynamics. The Person and Family Action Drawing can be done at the beginning of each session with the child. This diagram is essentially a blank piece of paper (landscape orientation) with the phrase "Draw A Picture of You and Your Family." Thus, there is no interpretation that something is right or wrong, everything is brought to it spontaneously by the client.

The following Figs. 2-4 and 2-5 beginning on p. 42 contain examples of an 8-year-old female victim of domestic violence and a 15-year-old male witness of domestic violence:

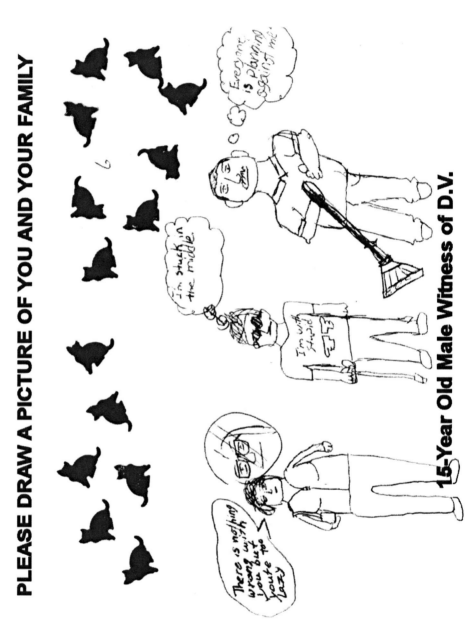

Fig. 2–4: Person & Family Action Diagram /15-yr Old Male Witness of DV

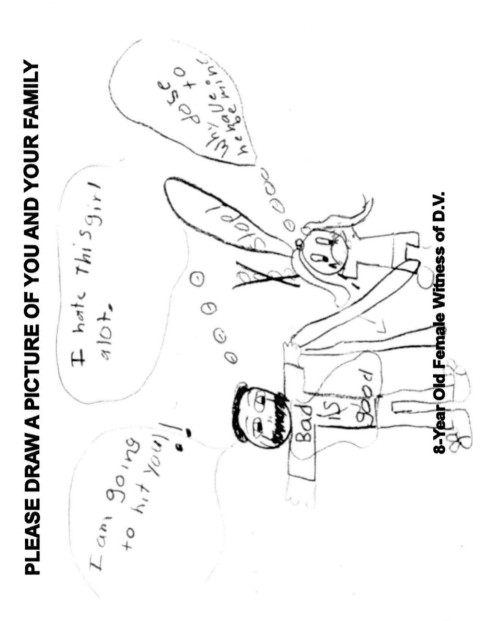

Fig. 2-5: Person & Family Action Diagram /8-yr Old Female Witness of DV

Basic Techniques for Children

In some cases, you may want to do some of these even before taking the child's history. These techniques help the child to feel:

- Safe with the counselor
- Safe being controlled
- Able to exercise self-control

Use any combination of the following before TIR or Unblocking

A. Explore:

Past experiences in therapy, particularly hopes and aspirations for the therapy compared to the actual outcome.

[Exploration refers to asking questions that do not have a preset pattern, but stay person-centered (in the sense that we mean it here), and stay on the topic being addressed. –Ed.]

B. "Do I remind you of someone?" If so:

1. "Tell me a similarity between _____ and me."
2. "Tell me a difference between _____ and me."

(Done as a 2 part loop: 1, 2, 1, 2, etc., to an end point.)

C. 1. "Look at that ____ (object in the room)."
2. "What is reassuring about it?" (Either make sure the child understands the word 'reassuring' or use a question s/he understands better such as "What about that _____ helps you to feel better?")

(Done with different objects, repetitively to an end point.)

D. "What is interesting about that _____ (object)?"
(Done with different objects, repetitively to an end point.)

E. 1. "Notice where you are right now." 2. "Spot some place where you are not." (Repetitively to an end point.)

F. "Look around here and find some action would be willing to take." (Repetitively to an end point.)

G. A three-part loop about safety.

1. "Tell me something it is safe to be."
2. "Tell me something it is safe to do."
3. "Tell me something it is safe to have.

(Three part loop to an end point.)

Misdeed Questions for Children: Theory

Use the following when directed by a supervisor. Generally, this list will be used when a child has behavioral problems and/or when a child is in a blaming mode.

To ensure that a child will participate, it is very important that you first let the child know that you won't tell on him/her. Remind the child of our reporting responsibilities, but other than that, we won't tell anyone. If something comes up that we think should be shared, we will encourage him/her to tell, with you present to help handle any parental reaction, but we won't force the issue.

Let the child know that you are going to ask a series of questions about things that s/he may have done. You can explain: "A lot of times, if you are angry, unhappy, and behaving in ways that hurt other people, it's because you've done things that you feel bad about. We're going to give you an opportunity to say these things and get relief."

Now, for each question, tell the child that you will ask what the question means and for the child to make up an example. After that, ask the child the question. Note the reaction, because if the answer is "no", but the eyes start shifting, or looking down, or in some way show a flinch, the likelihood is that the answer was "yes". In that case, ask if s/he is sure, remind the child that you're not there to judge, and ask again. If the answer doesn't change, leave the issue.

When a child answers positively, get ALL of the data: when, where, how many times, with whom, who doesn't know, who should know, and any other question that will complete the information.

If the child continuously answers negatively, try asking if s/he knows someone else who has done something like that. If so, get all of the data. At this point, ask if s/he's ever done anything similar. If so, get all the data.

Misdeed Questions for Children

1. Have you ever skipped school?
2. Have you ever hit someone first?
3. Have you stolen anything?
4. Have you ever broken something on purpose?
5. Have you ever painted on someone else's property or done graffiti?
6. Have you ever tried to hurt someone's feelings?
7. Have you ever lied to get someone in trouble?
8. Have you tried drugs?
9. Have you tried alcohol?
10. Have you ever smoked?
11. Do you own a weapon?
12. Have you ever used a weapon?
13. Have you ever hurt an animal?
14. Have you ever killed an animal?
15. Have you ever shoplifted?
16. Have you ever cheated on a test?
17. Have you ever successfully gotten revenge?
18. Is there something that your mother or father doesn't know about you?
19. Is there some question I shouldn't ask you?

Misdeed Questions for Parents/Caregivers

[Parents can develop critical, negative attitudes toward their children after doing them harm, either intentionally or inadvertently. Addressing these misdeeds directly helps a parent to clean these up and return to a more positive attitude toward the child or children in question. Fill in the blank with the child's name or as appropriate. -Ed.]

1. Have you ever hid something from _____?
2. Have you ever threatened _____?
3. Have you ever isolated _____ from the family?
4. Have you ever done something to get back at _____?
5. Have you ever asked _____ to do something s/he shouldn't do?
6. Have you ever ignored _____'s feelings when s/he's been upset or angry?
7. Have you ever ignored _____'s concerns?
8. Have you ever hit _____?
9. Have you ever shaken _____?
10. Have you ever cursed at _____?
11. Have you ever choked _____?
12. Have you ever pulled _____?
13. Have you ever pushed _____?
14. Have you ever thrown anything at _____?
15. Have you ever slapped _____?
16. Have you ever used a weapon against _____?
17. Have you ever tried to get _____ in trouble?
18. Have you ever stolen anything from _____?
19. Is there something _____ doesn't know about you?

3 | TIR & Art Therapy:
A Conversation with Anna Foley
as Interviewed by Victor Volkman

Victor: Tell me about using TIR along with art therapy in treating children.

Anna: Yes, I've kind of adapted both things to work together. I have training in both ways of working and I amalgamated them based on clinical need. I've worked for ten years in the field of trauma, six of those years as a practitioner with children in a victim support setting. This combination was the most effective technique I could use.

Victor: Tell me a bit more about your background.

Anna: I initially trained in Play Therapy and part of my clinical placement in 1993 was to work at the University of California Medical School in San Francisco. During that time, I did a three month internship and met Linda Chapman, an art psychotherapist who was based at San Francisco General Hospital. She ran the art and play therapy program there; she is board certified with the American Art Therapy Association. I asked her if she would take me on for the next year with my training and I returned again the following year. It was here I learned her neuron-developmental art therapy technique. After TIR training, I decided to go to King's College medical school and obtain more art psychotherapy training. I graduated from that program in 2001.

Victor: When you get a child referred to you, how do you go about deciding which procedure to use after the intake?

Anna: Usually I do a symptom checklist, with the family as well, not just with the child. I give all members of the family a chance to tell me what they think is going on. The family usually tells me what's changed with the child in their view, and how they feel they have changed themselves. It usually transpires that they are able to identify why they are seeking help at this point. Victim support is very different from a general clinic because you can get children referred quite quickly after a trauma. After a stabbing or a gunshot wound, you might see them in a week or within a month, whereas with a child in a clinic, you've got longstanding problems to deal with. In the interview, I try to ascertain how severe the symptoms are.

Victor: In a typical session, how do the various methods fit together?

Anna: I do some psychoeducation about trauma and the technique for the whole family. I use images to show how stress, traumatic stress or otherwise, can affect ordinary functioning. Mostly, families come to me when they have got beyond their normal coping mechanisms. Often I just get going. Children just want to tell their story, and get on with it. Lengthy assessment is counter-productive in these cases. I basically do a TIR session using images. Each session, I convey that it's a normal reaction to an extraordinary and painful experience. It's an ordinary reaction to an extraordinary event.

Victor: Right, so there's nothing "wrong" with them, that's just how life works?

Anna: Absolutely. Despair can be alleviated by normalizing symptoms. I feel that once that despair is alleviated, they have the opportunity to make an informed choice to then accept the art psychotherapy/TIR intervention. Before then, they are just a bundle of symptoms and I don't feel that it's properly an informed choice at that point. It would just be a desperate attempt to feel better.

An important thing for me as a practitioner, particularly in the field of trauma, is being able to be the person who can contain the horrors that the child and family have experienced. It is imperative to hear it, contain it, and alleviate at least some of it.

Victor: Good point.

Anna: Once I've done that (psychoeducation) and I can see that there's some recognition of what I'm talking about, that's usually when most family members are nodding and saying "That's what it's like." Then I can ask them, "Are you ready to go to the next stage?" I know there is some debate about long assessment or not, but I find alleviation of the arousal is of utmost importance. In a sense, background assessment can be put together during treatment. That's my invariable practice. The first session is to give hope. The art psychotherapy method I use is influenced by TIR. I would have to say the real inspiration comes from both techniques. I wouldn't say I was applying TIR by itself and I wouldn't say I was applying art psychotherapy on its own.

Sometimes I don't ask the child, "When did the incident begin?" because over the past ten years I've found that children make so many assumptions and connections about that day's experience that there might be something that pre-dates the incident itself. With TIR, we might find that out later, but to help them sort things out quickly, I actually ask them to start the image-making at the beginning of that day; what their first memory was.

I tell them at the outset that the way that it works is almost like going through a comic, where each memory is stored in a pictorial freeze frame form. If you've got lots of pictures, then it's a little bit like a comic strip in your head, or like a movie. They usually say, "Yeah, it's exactly like that and I can't stop it running, it's too scary!" So I say to them: "I want you to make the picture exactly like you've seen in your head." Each piece of paper is a different scene. So that might take 30 pieces of paper, it might take 40 to 50, or as few as 10. But whatever it is, it's right; it can't be wrong. Whatever they have drawn, we map that out so one piece of paper reflects each memory.

Victor: When you come to the end of the incident, you just know it because they put down the pencil?

Anna: Basically it's very much like being a TIR facilitator in that sense. All I'm saying is, "What happened next?" I'm acknowledging: "Good. You've done that image, now what happens next?" and I turn the paper. I take that piece of paper and I stack them in their order and go straight on to the next image. They very rarely pause; the only time hesitation comes into the image-making is when you get really to the most charged part of the incident. It starts to fluctuate, so I know, "Aha, we're getting to the bit that's probably causing the biggest problem." That's a very telling indicator.

Victor: They might start drawing slower or show some emotion?

Anna: When you get to the charged part of the incident, you can very often see their heart beating through their clothes. You might see that they have clammy hands or that their eyes will dart from one side of the page to the other, or they might freeze. They might ask, "OK, where can I put this?" So I can see that they know what this image is, but actually externalizing it and putting it out into the world is really quite difficult. Out of all of the children I've worked with in the past ten years, I've experienced only one person who hasn't managed to actually get this bit of the image out. I don't think that lessens the effect of the technique, it's just that it's about choices. We still know that there's something to talk about.

Victor: Typically, how long would it take to go from first image to the last once?

Anna: I would say typically in instances where adults are having quite severe post-traumatic symptoms, the first run-through can take as long as an hour and a half. Even with children, I would always schedule an extended session as you would do with TIR. We do it without any talking during the first viewing of the incident. I ask them to only draw it and not even to say what's happening. So they're drawing only: they're accessing how it's stored and I think that's very useful. The second time we go through and I ask, "Can you tell me what happened?" At that point, what I do with children is that if they say, "Well, I was standing here and there was a bus coming along this way at this point," then I ask them, "Are there any smells you can remember?" and "Are there any colors you can remember?" So in that sense I help them build a picture and sometimes we can find things that have more charge than we might have known. I'm not suggesting or interpreting, I'm simply wondering out loud, to elicit the full story.

Victor: You're making a point not to interpret, such as "This red blotch means you're afraid of blood" or who knows what?

Anna: Absolutely not. I can see by talking to them about it, because usually it's a very simple drawing. It might be a box for a house or a school, usually stick figures for people. It doesn't matter how good the drawing is, just how it comes out is the important thing. I'm looking to find out what's happening at every sensory level. "What did you hear?" "What did you feel in terms of physical senses?" or "What did the carpet feel like?" in the case of someone has an experience of rape. I find that they will remember the wallpaper; they will know what the color of the carpet was or what the smells were. I'm asking them to help embellish the picture and improve their recall, and in turn improve their likely success of becoming symptom-free.

Victor: The first time through, they do the drawings and the second time through you ask them what happened here and what happened there and so on?

Anna: I ask them what was the first thing that happened that day and we go on from there with the "What happened next" questions. They might start off by saying "Well, I was tying my shoes," or "I was having my breakfast" or whatever. I just ask in a very factual way on the second time through, what actually happened. We're turning the pages over as we're going through each scene. In art therapy I was taught that the third time through I should ask how they were feeling. However, I've found over the years that children have so many connections between what they are thinking and feeling that now I ask them for both and then they can answer it really well. They make the most amazing connections between thinking and feeling.

One little 7-year-old boy was going through an incident where his bicycle had been stolen and he had been really badly beaten. I asked him the first thing he remembered at the beginning of that day and he remembered lacing up his shoes. So the picture was a big image of just his trainers [gym shoes]. I thought, I wonder what is the significance of that? It might be nothing. Sometimes it is nothing, but for him as he was tying his shoes that morning, he felt that something really bad was going to happen that day.

Victor: How do you handle end points?

Anna: It generally finishes easily in the sense that we have to get to the last image. Usually, their shoulders drop, their symptoms of arousal have abated. Most often there is a sense of relief and they give me a lot of eye contact by that point. When the really scary bits are discharged, they look at me as if to say "I've been through something," or "I'm starting to feel better," and I can acknowledge. It's at that point where they get relief.

We call this a "flat point" if there is still more to be dealt with, but the person has gotten through a good chunk of it and feels better. After that I'm looking for what I call the "debris", the bits that we haven't picked up that are connections with the experience rather than the actual experience. I do continue to use the technique in the next session. On the basis of what we might have missed, we might need to go through it again.

Victor: Do you do a follow-up in a week or so and find out how they're doing?

Anna: Usually yes. I operate with a package really. I say it's never less than six sessions, just so that the family and the child are informed as to what I think it'll take to make sure that it's OK. I'm not suggesting that it has to be that or it can't be more.

Victor: If you find an earlier incident that's tied in, do you make a note of it and come back later?

Anna: I take note if it pre-dates what they've been referred to me for. If symptoms are not abating, the next time I see them, then we will address that earlier incident. That's been very effective.

If an image is made about a feeling that is really unmanageable, and we've looked at it and talked about it, I can ask, "How do we actually change the picture to improve things?" I've found that very effective. It's very interesting when children make new images of something that's really scary and dangerous, and then afterwards their brain cannot remember it again in the same way. Once I feel that they're ready to do that kind of thing, and although we have desensitized the actual incident, there's still something... you might not be able to shift a smell from under your nose or remove a picture from your brain. So, what I then do is to work on that image. For example, if they just have an image of an attacker's face recorded and it's not really attached to anything, then I ask them, "Well, how could you change that?" Usually they will go for it as well and they might make a really scary person's body into something funny like a clown or a fairy.

Interestingly, there was one case of a child who had witnessed a burglary and had not recovered in nine months. (His symptoms were not abating). He had seen this person in his house and he was very, very scared. He changed this guy's picture into something quite ridiculous: part "Spice Girl" and part animal. I checked on him again a week later and the man's image had faded from his memory.

Victor: That reminds me of a creative procedure my wife uses once in a while: "run them over with a steamroller" or "drop them into the ocean," etc. *[In a situation where someone felt powerless, this sort of creative technique allows the client to discharge pent up fear and anger through the use of imagination. It brings about laughter and relief. – Ed.]*

Anna: Yes, absolutely. That's a technique I also use. When the post-traumatic symptoms have become almost traumatic in themselves, as in revenge fantasies, I ask them to do that. Let them have the revenge fantasy and have it in a really safe way. They might have them hung up, or starved in the woods, run over, or actually shot, or other things that they can't really do. That's empowering for the kids.

Victor: What is the typical age range you work with?

Anna: Usually from age seven all the way up to eighteen. Below that you can use it, but it has its limitations. I worked with a 5-year-old girl who had witnessed a murder, and drawing ability as a way of mapping it out wasn't really available to her. It was OK because we were able to set out toys and ask, "Well, what did the scary person do then?" and use the same sorts of questions: "What did you hear?" and so on. "What were you thinking when you heard the screaming?" (Of course the child thought she was going to be killed).

Victor: You're using play therapy at that point?

Anna: Yes, but I'm doing it in a more directed way. You can work with children in the traditional model of play therapy in an undirected way, but that's less useful with trauma.

Victor: How has TIR improved your effectiveness with children?

Anna: It's been invaluable to me. I trained in TIR in 1994 and I've never stopped using it. TIR permeates every technique that I use and it's the backbone of what I do. The training was incredibly rigorous and opened my eyes to lots of things. It actually made me feel that I was able to take on more as a practitioner than I thought I could. The knowledge I've gained with TIR in the background helps me with all of my relationship work as well. After having it in my life for 10 years I can't really separate it out. My training was thorough and gave me an excellent appreciation of the predicament of traumatized children and adults.

4

The Value of Material Objects for Clients in Session:

By Marian K. Volkman

Many established therapies use physical objects (which can include the client's own body), spaces, and activities in the course of the work. Art and dance therapy are used with both children and adults, while play therapy and sand tray therapy are most often used in working with children. (For the best book I know on play therapy, see *Healing the Hurt Child* by Donovan & McIntyre.)

Of course, in the subject of Applied Metapsychology, we have a method of working that utilizes what we call *objective techniques.* These involve the client moving around, observing, touching, and sometimes moving things in the physical environment. There is a whole body of theory behind these techniques that I won't get into here, but in this article I would like to explore the use of objects the viewer can touch and handle while doing subjective work.

People have asked me whether clients don't sometimes use playing with objects to distract themselves from the vital work to be done, but in fact, that is an entirely different matter. A client who is using objects in the environment as a distraction has actually become disengaged from the work some time before. Care and time must be taken to reestablish rapport between viewer and facilitator, and reengage the viewer before any effective work can be accomplished. In this chapter, I am talking about a different phenomenon, where the use of objects helps to facilitate the client's ability to view charged material.

I like to keep a number of interesting objects on the shelves next to my viewer's chair and have often observed that clients of all ages like to pick these up and play with them as they talk. (This very rarely happens during TIR and is much more likely when a viewer is doing Exploration and other lighter techniques, sorting thoughts, perceptions and feelings.) After interviewing a number of facilitators who also keep objects handy and observe beneficial effects when their clients make use of them during a session, I decided to delve into the matter and get more understanding of what happens.

It seems that there are three distinct reasons why having such objects handy can be useful to a client who is working in the context of subjective techniques: *expression, focus, and grounding/comfort,* which shade into each other. More than one of these functions may be combined in one session, but let us look at each one separately.

Expression

Let us start with *expression*, since that is the most similar to the therapies mentioned above. It was a new thought to me when Elina Falck (a TIR colleague in the Vancouver area), told me that inarticulate clients, who have trouble expressing themselves emotionally and verbally, can do much better if they have clay to work with or something else of a physical nature to manipulate as they talk. [Some people find it difficult to express thoughts and feelings in words, but are more visually and kinesthetically oriented. Certainly, it makes sense that they might find it more helpful to express themselves by using visible and touchable objects. Of course, in play therapy and art therapy, the activity is deliberately being used as a mode of expression for the client. Just having objects there and ready to hand as a viewer does subjective work without having the facilitator direct his/her attention to them allows this activity to be purely person-centered. It is then the viewer's choice whether to pick up the objects or not, and how to use them or play with them.

Focus

In the realm of *focus,* we are talking about the ability to direct attention and this is a problem for some people. Dr. Gerbode uses the term "cognitively literate" to describe someone who is able to move at ease through his/her mental world, to identify things and patterns within it, and to move them around. This requires the abilities to focus, to identify things, to see similarities between things and also to see the differences. Cognitive literacy is impaired without a good ability to focus. Many people, both children and adults, struggle with a combination of characteristics which has been labeled Attention Deficit Disorder. This can make viewing more difficult. In the opinion of many professionals, ADD/ADHD is grossly over-diagnosed. Whether or not someone suffers from an actual disorder, having objects to work with can be a stabilizing factor. For many it seems to allow them to gain more control over the focus of their attention and makes subjective work easier to do and more effective than if no objects are available. Such people often habitually play with their hair or pick at their fingernails, but external objects seem to be more satisfying and useful.

Another theory has it that some people are much more concrete thinkers and others are more abstract thinkers. The latter might be able to juggle abstract concepts with ease, while concrete thinkers might do well to have some visible, touchable, movable objects to help represent their thoughts while doing subjective work.

Comfort and Grounding

In TIR work, we use grounding if needed at the end of a session, especially if the client has worked hard and is at a flat point, but too tired to go on and may not be fully back to the here and now. Grounding facilitates reconnecting the viewer to the present moment and the physical world before the end of the session, something that usually just naturally happens if you are able to take the action to its full end point.

Some viewers may feel the need of a bit of grounding at various points in a session. If touchable objects are available, viewers often ground themselves by picking them up. Grounding and *comfort* are closely related. We know the value of balancing the negative with the positive in viewing. In fact, a lot of what a viewer does in session results in a reduction or dissipation of that mental mass and impacted energy that we call *charge*. Getting rid of charge is certainly a good thing, and much to be desired, but even so, that dissipation can leave an empty feeling. A client who is allowed to play with physical objects will often spontaneously repair that empty feeling. The new empty space left in the viewer's mental world as a result of reducing charge needs to be reordered to the client's satisfaction. For many people, having objects to play with provides comfort and grounding at the moment when the person most needs it.

It was really by accident that I became interested in these phenomena. I had fossils, shells and polished rocks on my shelves because I like to have them. My clients have taught me the value of having things there to look at, touch and move around as they spontaneously picked these things up or arranged them in different ways while they talked. I had two young boys coming to me as clients some years ago. One was quite articulate but the other hardly talked at all.

I had a hunch about bringing something over to the table (which I did between his intake interview and first regular session). It is a marvelous toy made of little diamond shaped bits of metal on a base that is a strong magnet. Sure enough, my nonverbal client played with that thing all through his sessions and it did seem to facilitate his viewing.

Now that it lives on the table, almost every client of every age plays with it at some time or another during sessions. The magnet is in a wooden frame about 12 inches (25 cm) across.

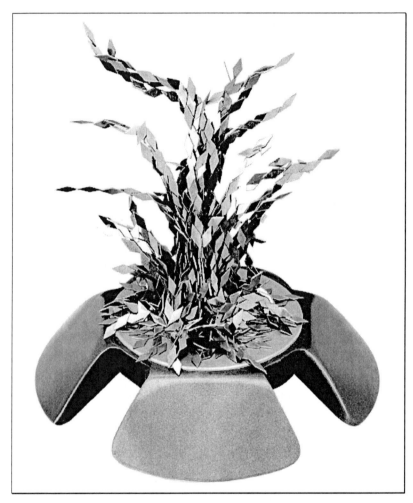

Fig. 4–1: The "Magnetic Feel", A Magnetic 3–D Sculpturing Toy

The "Magnetic Feel" (pictured above) is an example of the same sort of desktop toy that can be used over and over again in many creative ways. The original version is called the "Magnetic CRDL". You can find several sources for these on Google or eBay. The advantages of a magnet-based toy vs. clay, for example, are that clients won't get their hands dirty while working with it, and it will last practically forever.

<table>
<tr><td>5</td><td>

Future TIR: A Gift to Anxious Children who Have Experienced Traumatic Stress

Patricia A. Furze, MSW, RSW
</td></tr>
</table>

Working with children for over nine years in a mental health area of a local hospital, one of my challenges has been in assisting children to face a traumatic stressor. Once the need for this was acknowledged, it could be addressed and released. Future TIR a variant of Traumatic Incident Reduction developed by Marian Volkman, offers anxious children a focused, efficient way to process their fears of anticipate negative events[1]. These feared events are often projected into the future by these children. This chapter will explore this variant, how it has been used with children, the tremendous impact it has had on the resolution of traumas and how it's been used in preparation for other TIR sessions.

Children who have suffered trauma often experience symptoms of: varying levels of mood instability, sleep difficulties and disorder, interpersonal difficulties, eating and elimination difficulties, focus and concentration struggles, and behavioral difficulties. Often the mood instability occurs as depression or high levels of anxiety and panic. An overall increased sensitivity to others and the environment leaves them feeling vulnerable, exposed and out of personal control in their behaviors.

Anxiety is a healthy physiological response in our nervous system that alerts us to perceived danger. When we are anxious, a set of chemical and neurological responses occur, leaving us prepared for fight/flight, or freeze. For children affected by traumatic stress, the nervous system goes into overdrive and there is perceived danger in what seems to others to be innocuous events or circumstances. This stimulation of the nervous system leads many children (and adults as well), to become stuck in their responses, and less flexible. Procrastination and avoidance behaviors surface in the individual's attempts to self-manage and to decrease the fear of the unexpected.

One aspect of Western cultures that contributes to children's avoidance of unpleasant feelings and sensations is our instruction to children to use distraction to move their attention away from whatever upsets them. This works well in the short term. Repression pushes the

---

[1] Future TIR is a technique taught in the TIR Expanded Applications course (see www.TIRtraining.org)

sensations and feelings out of conscious awareness. They lie dormant, yet in a position to continue to affect the choices the child makes.

As a result of these factors, some children resist revisiting the traumatic events or experiences, but are willing to discuss in detail their fears of the future. These fears of the future often involve numerous cognitive distortions. Depending on the age and developmental stage of the child, they can also include some fantasy material. Imagined future events also have imbedded within them aspects of original traumatic events or experiences. According to Frank A. Gerbode, M.D., "TIR handles the negative feelings that cause people to have unwanted aversions to things." (Volkman, V. 2005)

For such children, Future TIR is an amazing resource. I have found these formerly reluctant and fearful children to more readily agree to and engage in Future TIR. It works well on events that are likely to occur as well as those unlikely to occur. A person's ideas about a dreaded future event can contain fixed beliefs and irrational fears, which lose their intensity and become desensitized and benign through the application of Future TIR.

When working with Future TIR we start with the worst possible scenario that the person (child or adult) could imagine as the first version to address. With some exploration, a time period is determined to establish some parameters and to identify a starting point. Each version is viewed until the child is no longer interested in it. At this point the child imagines a version that is slightly better and continues viewing again and proceeds with progressively better versions. The child indicates readiness to move to another version through interest in that version, or lack of interest in it.

During this work, the client can become aware of existing or new avenues of possible support and resources. The session completes when the child is no longer troubled by the originally feared event and circumstance. Often the child is more relaxed and feels more capable of handling the dreaded event. Change becomes less scary and more possible. Resilience often increases and the child develops enhanced emotional and cognitive flexibility.

Here are some examples of the myriad ways Future TIR has been used with children from toddlers to young adults.

Michael – Fear of Tomorrow

Michael, age ten, presented as a very emotionally unstable, somewhat immature, sensitive, child, large for his age but highly fearful.

Since grade one, he had experienced ongoing incidents of name-calling, and ridicule. Over time, the verbal taunting had escalated and had become physical. He was being pushed, poked and tripped. Michael had received speech therapy intervention as a young child and never felt confident that he could express himself verbally. He retreated into himself, trying to make himself invisible to avoid being noticed. However, his size and his tendency to cry and withdraw made that difficult to achieve.

At the point he came for assistance, he was shunning all social contact and was being bullied by a number of children on a daily basis. His increased reactivity and suspicion of others made it difficult for children to support him. He was very isolated and lonely. Michael alluded to an event that occurred in grade one that had been the start of his difficulties, but was unwilling to discuss it. He was willing, however, to discuss his numerous fears about what lay in store for him at school the next day. Over the next couple sessions, Michael was introduced to TIR and to the variant Future TIR and readily agreed to try it. He was having ongoing stomachaches, calling parents to request they take him home, and dreaded going to school.

He fit the profile of a child who can slide into school avoidance, and to curtail this we decided to move to Future TIR as quickly as possible. Michael cautiously began his session and once into the first of several scenarios, he fully immersed himself in the process. He ran through the first scenario three times, and then was asked to make it slightly better. What came next was a qualitative shift, as if Michael was now recounting the experience of the grade one event. He continued with this next scenario seven times, becoming progressively less tense, expressing lots of tears, shame for the action of others and becoming calmer. He was asked to create another, better scenario, and did so for two repetitions followed by a big sigh of relief and a smile.

At the next session, Michael's mother was jubilant in recounting Michael's shift. He was now able to leave for school more easily, he had not had any bad dreams over the week, and he had not called home asking to be picked up from school. Michael's teacher had noticed a difference in the classroom; he was projecting a more confident manner.

Michael met me with a big smile and a more relaxed demeanor. He spoke about how the other children did not seem to be bothering him. He reported his good news with more direct eye contact. He identified a couple of incidents that were still on his mind that he was now ready to address with TIR. He also began to talk about a future that could include friends and possibly having others to his home to play. Completing another thematic TIR session related to the bullying behaviors left Michael more aware of his contribution to the situations and a willingness to assume his own personal power.

Within four months, Michael was reporting no difficulties with peers. He could get perspective on the teasing he did encounter. Michael recognized that he was not alone, that others were teased as well. His problem-solving abilities increased. He was no longer triggered into feelings of shame and powerlessness. He started to reach out to others and saw himself capable of making positive things happen for himself and others.

Michael's school attendance became regular and his focus and concentration improved. His grades increased and he made one close friend and began to have play dates in his home. Michael continues to develop his social skills and to appropriately increase his level of independence. The Future TIR session seemed to have incorporated the incident from grade one and subsequently brought him tremendous relief.

Troy – Separation Anxiety

Usually unwanted feeling can be directly addressed with TIR, but sometimes a client's concern is so focused on the future that Future TIR is the best place to start. Addressing the dreaded future event can unburden that to the point where past incidents that were not previously accessible come to view. Troy, age eleven years, was able to use Future TIR to successfully address his intense anxiety when participating in sleepovers with his friends. He also eliminated his anxiety about being away from home on a school trip.

Separation anxiety often involves a shared avoidance of the fear of abandonment by the child and parent. When working with children who struggle with separation anxiety, the child is best supported by the therapist identifying the parent who shares the anxiety and involving that parent in addressing it too. I have found parents willing and receptive to engage in TIR sessions when they realize that they can assist their child through completing their own work. The following account involving Troy illustrates this process.

Troy is a very sensitive boy and is close to his mother. His mother had felt abandoned by her own mother, an addict who had struggled with alcohol and prescription drug abuse. When his mother became preoccupied with her own fears of abandonment, Troy experienced her lack of emotional presence as abandonment. With his future concerns discharged, Troy and his mother agreed to use TIR to address their shared fear of losing one another. The incident they chose to address was Troy's first day of kindergarten. Troy's processing demonstrated his acute awareness of his mother's pain and the fear in dropping him off for school. He found it confusing and alarming, contributing to his own insecurity and fears. The session unfolded quickly and easily to a good end point, leaving Troy calm and settled.

His mother's session began with saying goodbye to him in kindergarten and went back to a number of earlier similar incidents that involved the theme of the terror of abandonment. This was a much longer session and the gains were enormous. His mother was able to achieve closure on her separation from Troy's father, the death of her grandmother, and the repetitive events in childhood wherein her mother had emotionally and physically neglected her while acting out her addictions. The impact on Troy was immediate. He became less burdened emotionally, and was happier more often. He became less cautious and more spontaneous and seemed to be gaining confidence in developing a social life. At last point of contact, his mother continued to work on her significant trauma history with another therapist, and continued to make progress.

Future TIR has also been used successfully with social anxiety. Situations such as answering a question in class, approaching a server at a restaurant to order, answering the phone, planning for going on a holiday, and preparing to give a speech have all been handled with Future TIR with successful outcomes for the children involved.

Future TIR has been a welcome approach for children whose attention is fixated upon fears of future and are frightened and reluctant initially to face the past. For older children, the Unblocking technique can be effective as well. In my experience, however, Unblocking tends to be too cognitively challenging and slow-moving for younger children.

Definitions

Unblocking: A procedure in which a number of mental blocks on a certain issue are addressed repetitively until charge has been reduced on that subject. (See p. 176 for an overview)

Future TIR allows one to meet the child at the point their attention is drawn to. Resolution of future fears often brings a sense of safety and a higher level of trust of self, which translates into more confidence in the exploration of past events.

References

AMI/TIRA (2006). *Traumatic Incident Reduction Expanded Applications Workshop*. Ann Arbor, MI: AMI Press.

Gerbode, F.A. "Metapsychology: The Un-Belief System" in Volkman, Victor (2005) *Beyond Trauma: Conversations on Traumatic Incident Reduction, 2nd Ed.*, Ann Arbor, MI, Loving Healing Press, p 296.

Volkman, M. "Future TIR in Volkman, Victor (2005) *Beyond Trauma: Conversations on Traumatic Incident Reduction, 2nd Ed.*, Ann Arbor, MI, Loving Healing Press, pp. 66-68.

6 Empowering Parents and Caregivers to Effectively Deal With Childhood Trauma

This Chapter and Chapter 12 in Part Two, Results, give some outstanding examples of parents' success in using these techniques effectively with their children and some good emotional first aid remedies that parents can use.

Normally, such dual relationships are to be avoided. However, due to its highly structured nature, the work described throughout this book lends itself very well to situations where the client and practitioner have dual or multiple relationships; much better than would some traditional therapeutic models. The Communication Exercises and Rules of Facilitation discussed in the Introduction and mentioned in several chapters provide a framework of safety. That said, no one ought to take on such a dual relationship unless she or he feels confident in the ability to keep the roles clear and separate.

Techniques to Use with Small Children or Infants in a Medical Crisis Situation

By Jessica Hand–DeMaria

These are some observations I have made regarding infant trauma and objective techniques from our experiences with one of our children, Tom.

[Objective techniques are those that direct the client's attention to the physical world, rather than the inner, mental world. – Ed.]

The reality of an infant is based in attachment[1]. Forming and maintaining a bond with a caregiver is a fundamental aspect of an infant's world. Whatever is happening with a baby, separation from a primary caregiver during a time of stress can add or trigger trauma. A baby cannot survive alone. She knows that. *[We are using "she" here in general for balance, since the main part of the text refers to s specific male child. Of course this would apply to babies of either gender. –Ed.]* Thus, to her, survival depends on close proximity to the person she knows is committed to her survival. In general, and always during trauma, a baby depends on the presence of trusted caregivers. There is no "later" to a baby. She cannot know that anyone will come back when she is left alone for any length of time. Whatever the traumatic situation, there should always be a familiar person present with a baby or child. She cannot advocate for herself. Much that would be overwhelming and frightening becomes manageable when a baby knows the person who cares for her survival is present.

Tom was first admitted to the hospital at twelve days old. While his heart condition was diagnosed and he awaited surgery, Tony and I took turns sitting in a chair beside his bassinette. There was no way to hold Tom, and he was not sufficiently awake to make eye contact. It has been proven that a baby at birth shows a preference for the voices heard in the womb[2]. Tom was too young to know us on sight, but he knew the sound of our voices. We sang softly to him for hours. He

---

[1] For an excellent understanding of attachment theory, read *Becoming Attached* by Robert Karen.

[2] Laura Flynn McCarthy, "What Babies Learn In the Womb" in *Parenting Magazine*, January 1999.

seemed visibly calmed by our quiet singing. Even speaking to him had a definite orienting, reassuring effect.

Tom was so physically restricted and unstable during the weeks following surgery that we could not hold or feed him. Most of that time he was on life support and was rarely fully conscious. When he did open his eyes, it was a piercing, absorbed gaze that took in the whole environment. Our only way to maintain communication was simply to sit and lay a hand on his foot. The rest of him was covered with tubes, tape, gauze, and wires. Tony and I took turns, doing twelve hour shifts, sitting in a chair beside Tom for five weeks. During most of that time, we simply kept one hand on his foot, spoke softly to him, or dozed in a chair beside him. Even the simplest form of communication is stabilizing. I had feared that spending those weeks devoid of normal interaction would leave us strangers to him. However, the impact of maintaining simple continuous communication with Tom was remarkable. His preference for us was immediate. The moment he was "untethered" from all his tubes and wires, he curled up against us with utter apparent relief, clinging like a small monkey. If anyone else approached him, he cried and became tense and anxious.

After we went home, Tom was at an age when most babies begin to enjoy interacting with the environment. Tom had spent so much time overwhelmed by physical interventions and pain that he was reluctant to initiate any of the normal baby curiosity and exploration. He did not wave his arms, reach for objects, or try to roll towards them. Physically, he could do it, but he did not seem to know this. So, we thought of using simple objective techniques to help him feel present with the space. Objective techniques with a baby must be creative and based on whatever level of communication is real to him or her. So, with Tom fed and comfortable, Tony thought of a verbal communication we could try with him. First I got in good visual communication, lots of eye contact, just really letting him focus his attention on my face. When I felt he was present to me, I would make one sound: "Oh," or "Ah". I made one single sound, like it was the most wonderful thing I'd ever said. I would look at him expectantly. Often he would reflect back something with his face, raise his eyebrows, or pucker his mouth. I would acknowledge that with "Thank you!" Then I would say that sound "Oh," again as if it were the most wonderful sound in the world...just flowing all the joy I could flow into that sound. Typically Tom would begin to mimic me, and form a sound back. Of course, anything he did was joyfully acknowledged. We talked to Tom all the time. However, lots of sounds he couldn't copy had a different impact than a single sound he could manage. One single syllable would fascinate him. Sometimes, with practice, he copied my sound pitch perfect. He really knew he was being heard when I said, "Oh, wow, that is a wonderful sound!" It would start in his face and move all over him. He would clasp his hands and wiggle his feet and break into lots of smiles and puckers. He then began to make up "ooooh....ooh....AH!" sequences, in which *he* started to look at *us* expectantly. His whole presence became alert in the space, and his eyes lit up with curiosity and interest.

Another simple objective technique he loved was to have Tony take his feet, one in each hand, and move them in a little jogging motion. Tony had a silly song about "Running down the street, say hi to people I meet, and then JUMP the fence. I JUMP the fence." On the word "jump," he swung Tom's little feet quickly, carefully to one side as though he'd jumped over some pretended object in the way. Tom went wild over this. He lifted his arms and shouted little "ah, ah," gurgles and smiles.

At about ten months of age, Tom adored "Peek-A-Boo." He had a short medical procedure that month that required sedation. Tony and I always felt it was important to be present to comfort and orient Tom from the moment he came out of sedation. Imagine our amazement when he opened his eyes, looked at us, and said with a smile "Pyah boo!" He grinned with obvious relish over his joke. Two months later, after major open heart surgery, he awoke, gazed at us thoughtfully, closed his eyes, and said with careful finality "Key Ee Kah!" That was the last word he had learned before surgery: "Kitty Cat." Tony and I knew that was Tom's way of saying "I'm OK, I'm here, so don't worry." Tom was unconscious for 24 hours after he said that word. We would have been worried sick during that time. But we weren't. Tom picked the perfect communication to reassure us all was well. He knew.

During a very anxious day while he awaited that surgery, we ran several "empowering" objective techniques. A good woman friend of ours, Tom's guardian Angel, had let us know that during the ordeal, empowering Tom would be a useful response to all the overwhelming stimuli he would face. With that in mind, we passed the day prior to his surgery by inventing ways to give him a sense of control. He was te-thered to an intravenous pole and there is an eight hour restriction on food or drink before major surgery. Tom was miserable and refused to be entertained or comforted.

We found a small, soft ball in the gift shop. He was at an age where dropping something repeatedly was fascinating. Tony or I made a show of dropping the ball, while the other found and gave it back. We acted very serious and interested, and made a point of acknowledging the exchange of the ball from person to person. Tom was fascinated. We handed the ball to him. He immediately dropped it. Then he looked expectantly while we ran and picked it up. We gave it back. He was back in control! Just having a small ball to drop established communication and got him to be in the present. It was control he had lost, so it was control he wanted back. His emotional level (expressed through his eyes, facial expression, and general spirit) improved right away. I think we retrieved the ball dozens of times before he tired of the game.

Additionally, we had a little objective technique called "so strong". It was very simple. He pinched or nudged or squeezed our arm, and we appeared overwhelmed by his strength. "SO strong!" we would exclaim with absolutely sincere amazement. I went so far as falling straight down to sit on the hospital floor. He was feeling affected by his environment, so creating an effect himself delighted him. The bigger the effect he could create, the better. He was thrilled with the whole business. One good pinch, and mommy hit the floor proclaiming "So STRONG!" He thought it was fantastic.

We carried on like that all day until he fell asleep. Much of what would have registered later as overwhelming or terrifying was completely overlooked and forgotten.

The key to remember is that any benefit to objectives is entirely dependent on the parent being attached, attentive, and alert to the reality of the baby. Objectives can only work if the baby has a natural connection with the communication level used. I found that any interaction that fascinated Tom was a natural basis for objectives.

Never continue a technique past an end point. A baby knows when she is done with a communication. At all times and with all communication with a baby, always use her signals as your guide. Her sense of control depends on you paying attention and understanding his communication.

I found simple objective communication techniques to be invaluable tools that oriented and reassured Tom when he seemed to need more than the usual comfort of being held in a sling, rocked, or nursed. This was especially true during the times when he physically could not be held at all due to his medical condition and the treatment it required. These were very intuitive, "on the go" techniques, made up as we went along, based on what seemed real and interesting to Tom. What works to captivate and engage one baby may not help another. If you are a parent in this situation, build from your attachment, your love and knowledge of your baby. Pay attention. Read her signals. Babies know you are trying. They know when someone is there, to support and love and help them. Even when it seems there is nothing you can do to help your baby or to communicate, you are making a difference when you are simply present. Imagine yourself in a child's world, unable to speak, ask, or do anything for yourself. To know someone is there keeping an eye out, watching over and ready to assist, that is what makes the greatest difference to your baby.

Touch and Let Go

A Good, Fast Emotional First Aid Remedy By Renee Carmody

This technique is literally as simple as its name:

1. Facilitator: "Touch that _____." *(Points out and names an object.)*

2. Child: (touches object)

3. Facilitator: acknowledges, e.g., "Good," "OK," or "All right."

4. Facilitator: "Let go of that _____." *(Names object.)*

5. Child: (withdraws hand)

6. Facilitator: (acknowledges, as above).

7. Repeat until change in affect (emotional expression) upward on the Emotional Scale is noticed, or child loses interest or concerns.

There are two cases I remember off the top of my head where we used this technique. One was with a 12-year-old boy who had witnessed his father shot and killed while they were both at the family's business. The boy would not go into the room of his house where the father's portrait was hanging. I went to the home for sessions and had the boy touch and let go of his father's portrait. It was very difficult for the child at first, but by the end he was hugging his father's picture.

Another case was an 8-year-old girl who had nightmares about a monster. I asked her to draw a picture of the monster and then we went through the touch and let go until the monster held no charge. She stopped having that nightmare.

We find this simple technique very effective, especially with younger children who do not have the vocabulary to verbalize a traumatic experience.

Two Simple Remedies for Children

by Marian K. Volkman

Remedies are usually quite short techniques for times of stress when TIR would not be appropriate. Many of these are good for people of any age who are overwhelmed or distraught, who have been recently injured, or had something very upsetting befall them.

These two simple Remedies can be good for a child who has gotten hurt or doesn't feel well, and are handy first aid tools for parents. Even without any physical problem obviously present, you can do these to bring relief to a child who is generally upset. As with adults, we do not start or continue any technique without the willing participation of the person in question.

One of the problems in working with children is that adults often have a hard time believing that children can release the charge on something so fast. So be alert for end points, especially when doing light techniques such as these Remedies. A child's attention coming off what you are working on and on to the present environment can be mistakenly seen by adults as distraction or avoidance on the part of the child, when it is more likely to indicate an end point. A client's attention moving from an inward focus to freed up and moving outward onto the present moment and present environment is the key ingredient of end points. When in doubt ask, "How is that now?"

A few repetitions may be enough to brighten a child up, and that is a good place to stop, unless he or she is still interested in continuing. Going past that point of extroversion of attention will leave you with a child who may be unwilling to try this again another time. It's much better to do a little of each of these every day for a while with the child as a willing participant than to necessarily try to do everything in one session. Check for interest and willingness at the start of each session or each technique used.

Remedy A:

"Touch your ____ (part of body)"

Use your common sense. If a child has fallen and skinned a knee, you are not going to say, "Touch your knee," as that would be painful. You can say, "leg" and point to a place well above the knee for a few times and then switch to the other leg, and then eventually to a point on the leg below the knee. People trained in use of the **Touch Remedy** will recognize this as a simplified version. Remember to acknowledge (e.g., "Good," "Fine," "OK," etc.) for each task you ask a client to do.

Remedy B:

"Say hello to your _____ (part of body)."

It's a good idea to have the child say hello to parts that don't hurt as well as any that do. Direct the child's attention to body parts on both sides of the body. This is a gradient approach to the Communication with the Body technique that we use with adults. The end point is, again, that little brightening up and extroversion of the child's attention from whatever had been bothersome.

You can do both Remedies with a child consecutively, as long as you first do one of them and then ask the child, "Would you like to do another one?"

By the way, there is no reason why you could not do these Remedies with an adult as well, especially if you are dealing with a person who doesn't have much of an attention span at the moment. As with all Remedies, first aid comes first, then the Remedy.

<table>
<tr><td>7</td><td># Some ABC's of TIR and Metapsychology with Children</td></tr>
</table>

7

Some ABC's of TIR and Metapsychology with Children

By James Logan, RCC

[James Logan is a Registered Clinical Counselor in British Columbia, Canada. –Ed]

In more than thirty years experience working with children and their families, in individual as well as group settings, I have both adapted and translated various behavioral, educational and expressive therapies in order to reach the youngest of my clients. I have achieved exciting results using Traumatic Incident Reduction (TIR), and the Life Stress Reduction techniques of Metapsychology, with children and their parents. It has been a gift to be able to take clients to places of resolution that would previously have taken several sessions more, and most probably without complete resolution. Life Stress Reduction protocols are effective and efficient. Traditional approaches potentially result in clients making changes although they tend to experience prolonged suffering and unnecessary symptoms of distress or dysfunction. I was fortunate enough to discover TIR and Metapsychology˙ at a time when I had reached a place where I needed new tools.

The Case of a Boy with ADHD

One example of a surprisingly successful outcome occurred with a 10-year-old boy who had been diagnosed with ADHD (Attention Deficit Hyperactivity Disorder) and was taking medication for the condition. He was excited to have his first group birthday party, but worried about its success. During the intake interview, he expressed concern about his upcoming birthday party. In Applied Metapsychology, we always put the client's interests first so I immediately acknowledged his concerns and abandoned the interview for the moment.

This little boy was so concerned that his invited friends might not get along, it was clear that we should handle this first. Instead, I employed a Life Stress Reduction technique known as "Important/Not Important" concerning his birthday party. *[A repetitive series of questions of the form "About ___ What is Important" and "About ___ What is Not Important" –Ed.]* He achieved a successful end point within 10 minutes and as a result we were able to finish the intake interview.

The following week, the boy shared with me that he felt completely resolved on the birthday party issue. He proudly told me how he had dealt with his previous fear. Specifically, he let each invited friend know in advance who else was attending. This was a breakthrough for him, given his previous level of concern. We celebrated his success as he told me that everyone came to his birthday party and they'd all had a good time.

Focusing Your Attention

The more experience you have working with children, the more it boosts your ability to understand them. As you deepen your understanding of the theory of TIR and Metapsychology, it becomes easier to find the central elements to simplify the language in order to educate and guide even the youngest child through TIR and Metapsychology techniques.

The challenge for any TIR facilitator working with children is knowing the treatment modalities well enough to educate the concerned parent(s), and to be able to demonstrate the language you will be using to meet their child's age and stage of understanding. Working with children requires vigilance throughout the session to hold their attention while maintaining focus on their various needs.

To achieve or sharpen your 'child-focused' knowledge and experience, try working with your own children, or children within your extended family, or those of friends. *[Special care must, of course be taken in working with anyone, adult or child, with whom you have a dual or multiple relationship. See also the Introduction and Chapter 6 – Ed.]* Volunteering in educational or recreational settings will also lend opportunities for focus, interaction, and observation of children. Two key ingredients when working with children, as well as adults, are to listen and to show genuine interest in them.

In the Traumatic Incident Reduction training materials, *interest* is defined as directed attention. Communicate with children while deliberately focusing your attention on them. This ensures a powerful, positive result. Tap into your own curiosity about them, and be willing to see the world through their eyes. Children are quick to discern if you are not 'real' and authentic, and will react accordingly. Do all your work in a manner consistent with the child's age level. Find out how your child clients react to their own emotions, exciting activities, and the things they are passionate about. Sometimes children's reactions will be subtle and their thoughts or ideas may bounce around from one topic or idea to another.

They may move their talk away from topics that are too emotionally charged and close for them. They may at times avoid conversations completely. It simply means they are not yet ready to talk about the issue, and you must never force them into talking about it. In such cases, simply note their responses in addition to the content of their communications. There may be an opportunity to approach an area at a later time. Still others will show only a light degree of interest and then move on to a different topic. Often, the new topic will highlight a shift in their thinking or attitude, and in some cases may actually be evidence of an end point.

Creating A Safe Space

Throughout TIR, both children and adults need to feel safe. The Rules of Facilitation guide us to be genuinely attentive. *[See the Introduction and glossary for more on the Rules of Facilitation and the Communication Exercises. – Ed.]* A TIR Facilitator is trained to have a neutral attitude, to be non-judgmental, listen with interest, and be non–reactive to the content of whatever the person is working through. I personally have known clinicians who were not trained in the use of TIR—who did not have the benefit of practice using Communication Exercises, and who reacted to their client's story through some personal need to show empathy, or gasped at the recounting of details, all of which inevitably had a significantly negative impact on the client's outcome.

In addition to the natural human tendency to seek approval from others, children are often taught to seek approval from adults, since children are dependant on adults as their providers of emotional safety and basic needs. They will react internally to the ways people do or do not accept what they are communicating. It can be difficult to observe their true feelings, as children may continually be adapting to (or withdrawing from, or rebelling against) adults as they perceive how an adult wants them to act. This makes the mastery of Communication Exercises vitally important. They ensure that at all times you provide focused, directed attention with timely, fitting acknowledgements for the child client. It is essential throughout the child's work in the session that the facilitator is not perceived as being evaluative or judging, as this will shut down the viewing process. This is somewhat like those times when you might be listening to a child while driving your car. You may not hear the same content from the child when sitting face to face with them, so you strive to be as transparent as the windshield, which allows them to feel uninhibited and you to hear the information.

During work with TIR, the child quickly learns that it is safe to say anything, and that any thoughts are welcomed by the practitioner. Once this safety is established, children express what they want to, rather than what they think you might want to hear. This further encourages spontaneous child responses that access their subconscious. Emotional charge is thus reduced, leading to meaningful cognitive shifts for the child. Speak to the child in age-appropriate language. Be aware of and use the child's exact wording wherever possible. This approach includes nonverbal communications such as playing out themes, communication through expressive arts, and description of attitudes or emotional shifts, all of which can facilitate getting to an end point, which occurs when the child experiences success in resolving an issue.

Client As Expert of Their Own World

Applied Metapsychology asserts that clients are the best experts about themselves and no one knows their own subjective experiences better than they do. Humans instinctively know what they need in order to be healthy and be functioning at their best. However, the road to emotional freedom is not necessarily within their conscious awareness. I have had brilliant clients over the years and it has always been my desire to discover a method where clients can do their work in a way that parallels their own unique mental world. Some clients are able to locate and align with their own unique viewing material while working independently within their own unique mental environment. Through facilitation of Traumatic Incident Reduction and other Life Stress Reduction techniques, I have had the privilege of witnessing these clients achieve maximum results. TIR is a highly respectful approach facilitated by the practitioner, but guided by client interest. I simply provide the safety and structure to resolve traumas, facilitate the reduction of charge and acknowledge client resolutions and successes. The resulting actions by clients between sessions and the shifts in their lives surprise them, and those around them. It is common for cognitive shifts to continue between sessions. It is an ongoing and rewarding client-facilitator relationship.

Developmental Issues and Language

Certain groups of clients need the techniques to be described in simplified words. These include: English as a Second Language (ESL), highly charged, low literacy, or intellectually challenged clients, and especially, children. I have found it very helpful in making adjustments to accommodate the child's age and level of understanding. For example, I change 'methodology' to 'methods', 'terminology' to 'words.' I strive to keep the same meanings but to simplify language.

Other than adapting the words, the techniques follow the same protocols as for adults. I keep gathering and adding new material as the client's awareness shifts, as upsets are recalled or experienced, and again, I always endeavor to present issues in the child's own words. I also record (in parentheses) any changes in affect/emotion (called in Metapsychology, indicators). This allows me to check with the child to address any other areas of charge and interest that have emerged.

While the techniques remain the same, be ready for the subtle and quick cognitive shifts that often accompany children's view of the world. Children generally do this sort of work faster, reaching quicker end points than adults do. Another difference is how children talk. This varies depending on their age, verbal skills, vocabulary and use of slang expressions. I have even had a 9-year-old boy whose communicated using only sound effects for 80% of his verbalizations. I accepted what he vocalized and asked for clarification when I needed it.

Getting in Communication

Quickly assess their comfort with direct eye contact. Sometimes children appreciate you getting down to their eye level, while others are more comfortable being allowed to come toward you. Some children may exhibit a temporary need for personal space and shy away until they warm up to you. Many children will intrude on an adult's personal space, so be prepared to gently redirect them, and secondly to instruct them about appropriate boundaries. Watch them carefully without staring. If the child presents as timid or shy, turn your eyes to something in the room so that you can still observe them in your peripheral vision.

On first meeting, talk about something of interest to the child: a doll or toy, a television or movie character that the child brings up or brings into the session, or something interesting in your office. Be observant and parallel the child's interest. If children don't volunteer it, ask them what they like best about a character, show or story. Let them be the experts. Even if you know about the story, listen to how they explain it to you. This will help with rapport building and with gauging their responses when you are asking interview or procedure type questions. Once they have begun to talk, they tend to flow with information about the things that are of interest to them. Stories that are light, as well as ones that are laden with charge, will come forth, in response to the interest you show. Most young children are eager to perform and have you be their audience: "Watch me, watch me!" They may want your undivided attention. Be genuine with your enthusiasm and focus your attention on whatever excites them. This not only creates a spirit of fun, it fosters cooperation and willingness to follow what you will be asking of them.

When working with young children, I tend to introduce the educational parts only as needed along with simple examples to clarify and try out the method. Children might not have much to say, but they quickly tend to grasp the various techniques. Therefore, when they appear to be comfortable with the procedure, just go with the flow but watch their indicators closely. Again, when educating children about the techniques such as loops [one or more questions asked in sequence over and over until an end point is reached], I might say the following:

> "I'll ask you questions to help you and you might have lots of ideas. I'll probably ask you the same questions many times. This will give you the chance to tell each of your ideas about that question."

Then, I might use an example to provide encouragement while making only necessary protocol adjustments as required.

Children Who Have Difficulty In Communication

On one occasion, when I worked with an 11-year-old who did not want to make eye contact (and I felt that she was withholding something), I carried on with the Unblocking and was met with resistance in the form of nonsense answers. Speaking to the child directly did not move things along, so I changed to a Memory List where, after a few minutes, I was able to acquire the necessary cooperation and returned to complete the Unblocking.

[For examples of Memory Lists, see Appendix A--especially the last list which is used in case of session difficulties. – Ed.]

In another session, I was able to guide an imaginative 4-year-old through Basic TIR, in which a single known event is addressed, while he pretended to be in a Time Machine which was a cardboard box. I could still see the child's face through a window in the box while following the steps for Basic TIR. I asked the question, "When did it happen? Go there in your time machine." He was able to follow the steps through a minor traumatic event by using this adaptation. Because he had found sitting face-to-face difficult, I had already arranged to sit side-by-side with this child. Eventually, he was tested and diagnosed with Autism Spectrum Disorder. TIR and Life Stress Reduction tools are very accommodating in that they can be adapted to fit the language needs of the young child, and are most effective with older children and adults when followed exactly as designed.

Matching The Pace

The following is an example of matching pace with the child, and how accommodating the protocols can be. I worked with a 12-year-old boy who was very slow to verbally respond. (In fact, he was the slowest responder I have ever known.) Although his mind and wit were quick, changes in his emotional expression and behavior were very subtle, requiring close scrutiny. In addition, he had a previous negative experience with a psychologist whose strategy or approach included challenging the child's response to questions. As a result, for years he had refused his parents' attempts to get him to professional help.

It was imperative that I wait positively and expectantly for answers to my questions. I rigorously matched his cautious pace and followed through with protocols to match the information he gave me to work with. I accepted and never challenged his, "I don't know" responses because he was hyper-sensitive about the acceptance of his answers to questions. I would simply move on to the next question. At times, it seemed he would give me an answer out of the blue, until I realized that he was still answering the *previous* question.

According to his mother, the boy had been doing little to contribute around the house other than sometimes helping a sibling play video games, or programming the VCR. During the interview, he indicated high interest and distress regarding emotional charge around his single-parent mother. Two years earlier (age 10), he had chosen to live with his mother rather than his father, whom he visited on most weekends. I constructed a case plan which included a program of techniques to be used to deal with charge and difficulties concerning his mother. At one point, I had to recover an earlier missed end point where the only visible change had been when his shoulders relaxed a half inch, which was all that showed that he was more at ease. I closed the session with a Memory List.

Nothing significantly observable by me had occurred in our session. However, a huge difference began to show up at home! This boy went home, and for the next week, initiated cleaning and packing family items to help prepare for their upcoming move. He also encouraged his siblings to support their mother. The mother was shocked. She hadn't asked him to clean, and she had never seen him use cleaning products or rubber gloves before—and he was doing a good job! I hadn't spoken with him about any of these possible contributions; how he felt about his mother, what he could do, or how to set up an action plan or establish goals.

I am clear that had I followed traditional counseling methods I would surely have gotten in this boy's way, complicated his efficient progress or positive result, and gone into an unnecessary parade of steps. Yet, by utilizing Life Stress Reduction techniques, he launched himself into action literally overnight! Probably, the change was not through changes in his cognitive awareness, but he was independently able to sort out the thoughts that were blocking a shift in awareness and becoming cooperative. The main point is that I didn't need to know or guess what he was aware of for the techniques to work.

The Sand Tray

I use many media when working with children. One of their very favorites as well as mine is the sand tray. This is usually a rectangular container of 3:2 dimension ratio which varies from 8 to 12 inches deep filled half full with clean sand. The tray is on legs and should stand approximately waist high to the child for their ease in reaching items for play in the sand tray. There are various schools of practice that require a range of items for use in the sand tray. They generally include various animals, people figures, symbolic three dimensional representations, mythology items and props, fences, walls, trees, buildings and vehicles that are used to play out the themes, issues or storylines.

Even without language, there are representations of situations of family dynamics, conflicts and challenges through symbols and patterns of symbols. Children use the objects and I give them anything they ask for the scene they are creating in the sand tray. This is the child therapy equivalent of talk therapies with adults. Although sand tray work as a therapy with adults can sometimes be useful, it is less common. The setup for sand tray work is used to maintain the child's interest and is child-directed. This provides an opportunity for indirect/non-verbal interpretation by the therapist. It has its historical basis in psychoanalytic theory, but today there are many departures from psychoanalytic approaches. I have made use of sand tray work to create a dialogue with children and have had the experience of receiving either verbal or non-verbal responses played out in the sand tray.

Whenever appropriate, I have incorporated the sand tray along with the use of TIR and Metapsychology. This has proved to be effective when working with a child using Basic TIR. The sand tray is used to directly set up the beginning of an incident and continue to add new items or details that come into awareness. The sand tray can also be used as an intermediary with Life Stress Reduction questions, given that children often answer more easily when their hands are busy. Additionally, the creation in the sand tray may give me a non-verbal answer that wouldn't otherwise come forth. I take notes and make sketches of the sequences as the sand tray scenes develop for both verbal and non-verbal forms of response. I also like to photograph the sand tray work upon completion, which serves as an acknowledgement of end points.

Clay Work

With a quiet child, or one who is resistant to talking, I may introduce sign language as a way to maintain clarity for 'yes' or 'no' questions. Or, I may seek nonverbal responses by incorporating another expressive therapy such as clay work. Here we use non-toxic, non-drying modeling clay on a sanded piece of wood or clean table surface. The child can mold the clay into symbols, word balloons, or shapes that depict their answers, responses or solutions. As in the use of a sand tray, I sketch their representations along with my note taking.

The tangible, three-dimensional clay representations tend to have more significance to the older children (10- to 12-year-olds) I have worked with when using clay. Although it may sometimes be time consuming, there is often a much greater willingness in these children to engage with the clay than to provide verbal answers. TIR can lend itself well to the incorporation of art therapy media of expression using sand, clay, drawing or painting. Using these kinds of creative media with children can help to increase cooperation in situations where you may otherwise encounter reluctance or protest. Children love to make choices and you can use the opportunity to allow them to choose the medium that is the best fit for them.

The clay method also works well with the Metapsychology technique known as Exploration, asking many sorts of questions on a single topic while staying centered in the client's experience. For example, an 11-year-old child responded to the question "What has been happening to you at school?" by using clay to depict her answers of: "I'm not getting enough help" and "I don't want to sing in front of the class." What resulted were 3 columns of various clay representations much like the panels of a cartoon strip. As we continued to work through various clay representations, we incorporated different colors of clay to create distinctions between separate segments of the overall creation. The first column we devoted to "Feelings" and the child made clay models of the various feelings she had in connection with singing in front of the class. The middle column was devoted to "Alternatives." Here she looked at alternative ways of feeling to what she had been experiencing up to then. The third column was devoted to "Solutions." She modeled various solutions she could have for singing in front of the class. Within a forty minute session, the charge had been eliminated and the child no longer considered singing in front of the class a problem. To complete this type of session using a physical medium, I first have the child scrunch up the clay from the charged "Feelings" (left column), second the "Alternatives" (middle column) and finally, after reviewing the "Solutions" (right column) have her put away the clay.

Summary

I have found that TIR and Metapsychology protocols and methods always work best when accommodated to fit the needs of the child. This is especially true when using art media with children who had suffered trauma before the development of speech. Often a child does not have the vocabulary to talk about the traumatic events. However, we can let children depict their experiences through the use of colors, shapes, detailed representations, stick figures, symbols, etc. When drawings are used, I place them in a binder with a page protector to create the order of earlier or later events. In this way, the drawings can be used as their starting point, and you can have the child draw another page as things change. The emotional charge is evident and observable in many ways during these expressive moments. It is evident from the intensity or facial expressions displayed while the child is creating an expressive scene. Children may also choose to animate their creations with noises or even express words. For the most part, I let them create and clarify any fine points they wish to add by asking unobtrusive questions. The key point here is not to interfere with their process, but to let them experience cognitive shifts on their own. I check for end points, wins, or things to clean up as circumstances dictate. Finally, I facilitate closure using grounding techniques (simple techniques used to drawn the client's attention to the present moment and surroundings) or Memory Lists.

I continue to be greatly impressed by the quality of the Metapsychology techniques, including TIR. Other counseling modalities and expressive therapies can benefit greatly by including the delivery of TIR and other Metapsychology applications with younger children. Children will reap the benefits of the seemingly magical outcomes and resolutions these techniques make possible. The remarkable generosity of my trainer, Brian K. Grimes, and the many people I have met as a result of my continued training and involvement with TIR have inspired me to share my talents and experience working with children. It is a privilege to be a contributing member of the growing collective intelligence of the international TIR community.

Part II:
Results

8 Two Examples of Detailed Case Studies Using TIR with Young People

By Patricia Furze, MSW, RSW

Strengthening Focus and Concentration Using TIR with an Adolescent Identified as Learning Disabled

This case report explores the life of a young woman who presented in crisis for assistance in the Mental Health Department at a local hospital. Unrecognized seizures and traumatic stress had a profound impact on her and she was identified as "Learning Disabled" by the Canadian school system. Traumatic Incident Reduction was used conjointly with family therapy and individual therapy to support her. In addition to other positive gains made during the treatment, the use of TIR appears to have unlocked the blocks to learning experienced by her.

Background

Linda was fourteen years of age when she arrived for an urgent appointment at the Child Mental Health area. She was having recurrent thoughts of harming others and was seething with anger. One of five children, Linda was becoming increasingly isolated. She found herself in conflict with friends and unable to tolerate what she viewed as the petty gossip of others her age. Linda felt aged beyond her years, given what she had experienced in her family, and found it difficult to relate to the backbiting and rejection that she found only too common with her peers. Linda also had little tolerance for lies and deceit and felt compelled to speak her truth. This often left her feeling like a "bull in a china shop" with others' feelings and was shunned as a result. Linda also felt despair over her diagnosis of Learning Disability in mathematics and English, and being sent to be with a small group of children for extra support. She and this group were viewed by their peers as "stupid" and subject to criticism and the humiliation of name-calling.

The exploration of Linda's history revealed a young girl born into a troubled family. The mother, a survivor of horrific intergenerational abuse, required intensive and ongoing mental health intervention. The father, amidst all of the psychosocial and financial stressors, developed severe colitis requiring ongoing medical attention. Linda was a middle child, primarily mothered by her elder sister. Despite her mother's dedication and investment in her own healing, Linda observed her mother being taken to hospital by ambulance after having overdosed on a couple of occasions.

In grade one, Linda began having *petit mal* seizures regularly (see Sidebar at end of article) which resulted in her feeling confused and spacey and missing significant content in the fundamental learning. It was not until grade two, when Linda had already experienced significant gaps in learning, that her seizures were noticed by a keen and sensitive teacher. At this point, Linda was given seizure medication which quickly controlled the seizures. This medication was withdrawn when Linda was in grade five and she no longer experienced seizures. By that time, she had been identified and tested for Learning Disabilities and had begun receiving supplemental support for math and English. Sadly, this help proved to have a dark side given Linda's needs, as she was teased and name called and felt that there was "something wrong with my brain."

While these challenges presented at school, home life was filled with severe marital conflict and the ongoing threat of breakup. When I met Linda for the first time, she had just overheard her father threatening to leave the family. Linda acutely felt both the terror of abandonment and rage.

In Therapy

During the first few months of therapy, Linda had to confront a fixed belief that you did not speak about family experiences to those outside the family. The family itself also had an operating belief that it was unsafe to talk about feelings inside the family too. As she explored these fixed beliefs, Linda recognized how maintaining them created feelings of isolation for all members within the family and with the larger community. Her fears that she would be judged, ridiculed and blamed were not realized in our therapeutic relationship. This support allowed her to gain some hope that things could change for her in a positive way. She focused on developing a clearer understanding of herself and of her role in the conflict emerging within her close friendship circle. Taking responsibility for her role without blaming and self-recrimination was challenging yet also liberating for Linda. As she gained new clarity and an emerging sense of her own power to make choices, she found the confidence necessary to explore her family life.

Linda agreed to family sessions, in order to begin to open up communication with her parents. She particularly wanted to let her mother know of the devastating impact her mother's own mental health struggles had been having on her. She wanted to tell her of her feelings of abandonment that were reawakened each time her mother withdrew from the family to manage herself. She also wanted to understand her mother's diagnosis and where she was in her treatment. She had noticed improvement in her mother's functioning after seven years of intensive treatment but knew that her mother continued to be volatile and at times required daily intervention.

This family session, attended by both parents as well as her mother's own therapist, went well. With the support of her therapist present, Linda's mother was able to discuss her diagnosis and the impact it had on her daily life. She spoke about her commitment to her healing and her love of her family. Linda was able to ask questions about her mother's trauma history, and albeit with some difficulty, her mother was able to share some parts of her history. One challenging question posed by Linda to her mother involved whether her mother believed that her own father (i.e. Linda's grandfather) had been a perpetrator of this extensive abuse. This challenging question allowed her mother to confront rather than deny this past reality. It became evident that Linda's mother had a deep love for Linda and for her children, but her sense of self had been severely shattered by her early and prolonged and repetitive physical and sexual abuse. Linda's parents were finally able to give feedback about her chronic rage and their confusion about how to interact with her and their wish to support her. Linda's father felt that for the first time he better understood his wife's mental health needs and treatment planning. He was able to take responsibility for the marital conflict and the impact it had had on the children. He was also able to discuss his own medical condition and the effect the prolonged stress and his struggle to manage it was having on his health.

Linda came away from the session somewhat confused about her positive although limited experience of her grandfather and her mother's broad report about the neglect and abuse experienced. She chose to speak with one of her aunts to gain her perspective as an older sibling to her mother. Although her aunt did not want to discuss it in detail, she was able to corroborate her mother's recollections. Linda tried to sort through the dichotomy in her experience of her grandfather as a quiet, somewhat ineffective man and the brutal abusive man who horribly injured her mother. She sought to understand how anyone could inflict such harm on their infants and young children. Linda found new compassion for her mother, seeing her as this vulnerable child. She was also non-judgmental, making the leap to wonder about the circumstances in her grandfather's life which would lead him to making such destructive choices. She requested literature to help her to better understand her family history. Linda explored what this meant for her view of God and of life in general. She also chose to discuss with her siblings her newfound understanding of her mother, her life experiences and treatment planning. Slowly Linda was establishing stronger emotional connections within her family.

TIR Results

For Linda, this family therapy session allowed her to focus on the impact of her parents' situation on her life and she committed to using Traumatic Incident Reduction to process her experiences. TIR was thoroughly explained and practiced on a non-triggering event to familiarize Linda with the procedure.

The first TIR session focused on her mother's suicide attempts. Specifically, we addressed an incident where Linda had witnessed her mother being taken to hospital and wondered if she would ever see her again. During this two-hour session, Linda confronted the feelings of abandonment and anger toward her mother and the family members who had victimized her mother. Her fears of somehow being responsible for her mother's suicide attempts surfaced. She addressed the jealousy she felt toward her mother's own therapist. Linda believed that her mother was more attached to her therapist than to Linda herself or any other family member.

During the session, she also went back to similar incidents involving earlier times in her young life when she had felt abandoned. This took her to the time when she was hospitalized for her seizures at age eight and had restricted visiting. This early experience occurred at a time when the hospital policy enforced limited visiting hours for children. This policy, combined with the multiple needs faced by her parents, had meant that she'd had little time with them while in hospital. Consequently, their absence left her feeling abandoned and bereft. However, she was now able to recall having had positive time with the nurses attending her, and could see how support from them and others in the community had helped her to feel connected and cared for.

This new level of awareness arising from her TIR experience allowed Linda to have more empathy for her mother and an appreciation for how important the support she received from her therapist was to her. Linda also was able to recognize the community support that was available to her, for example through the family's church, whose members helped out with clothing and in offering positive peer-programs. At the end of the session, Linda had desensitized the aspects of her anger and helplessness arising from all these incidents. She began to reflect on the support and care that also surrounded her, even though it had often come from individuals outside the family.

The effects of this single TIR session were profound and multiple. Linda became less emotionally reactive, she felt less guilt and shame and her self-esteem improved. She developed the strength to set boundaries in her friendships, which lead to a begrudging respect from her friends. She identified the need to develop assertiveness skills. Linda worked diligently at using an assertiveness protocol, practicing the skills, and reporting back on her success. Rapidly, the locus of control became internalized and she began to practice maintaining her own power. She learned that saying 'No' was an option and as she practiced limit-setting, discovered a new freedom to honor herself. Linda happily reported increased concentration and focus. Her memory improved and she appeared to be better able to integrate new learning. Contact with Linda's parents revealed that they were experiencing the positive effects as well. They noted that Linda was less angry and argumentative and communication had improved.

Linda's grades improved dramatically at school. One year post TIR she was getting As and Bs and two years post TIR she received Honors and was considering moving into an advanced level of course. These developments in her learning raised the question for Linda as to whether she had actually ever had a Learning Disability. She wondered whether the early missed learning caused by her seizures and ongoing high level of stress and low support had contributed to her irregular scores on the psychological tests for learning disability. She recognized that she benefited from the level of extra support by being identified as Learning Disabled. Given the general lack of support in her larger life experiences, this extra support was valuable, but she was aware that being identified "learning disabled" had also left her feeling different and damaged.

Linda again agreed to using TIR to process her feelings of inadequacy and torment over the name-calling and teasing she had experienced. She readily engaged in the TIR and again processed a number of powerfully negative interactions with her peers. The calm and peace she experienced at the end of her session became part of her social interactions. Her self-esteem increased and her ability to maintain a positive sense of herself grew. As she left high school, Linda graduated with

Honors and received a Scholarship. I recently encountered Linda's father at the local hospital and he beamed with pride telling me about Linda's success. She has now finished her social work degree and is committed to supporting other young people in their struggles to be all of what they can be.

Linda's experiences raised questions about whether the testing for learning disability had actually picked up missed core learning at the grade level, compounded over the years, creating gaps in learning fundamental to Math and English. Linda's seizures going unnoticed or perhaps misunderstood for about a year at such a critical developmental time certainly impacted on her memory, concentration, focus and learning. The school system in Canada had responded with support and assessment. Those involved had put in place a supportive plan for Linda, which was helpful to her, especially given her challenging home environment. As those in the trauma field recognize, early life traumatic experiences profoundly shape the development and life of those affected. It is my hope that early neglect and traumatic stress will be quickly recognized for its contribution to apparent learning disabilities.

Fortunately for those such as Linda who commit themselves to working through these traumatic events even long after the fact, focus, memory and concentration can and do improve. Individuals can and do go on to develop a positive and strong sense of self and to actualize their dreams.

A *petit mal* seizure is a temporary disturbance of brain function caused by abnormal electrical activity in the brain and characterized by abrupt, short-term lack of conscious activity ("absence") or other abnormal change in behavior. Petit mal seizures occur most commonly in children ages 6 to 12. They may occur in combination with other types of seizures.

Typical petit mal seizures last only a few seconds, with full recovery occurring rapidly and no lingering confusion. Such seizures usually manifest themselves as staring episodes or "absence spells" during which the child's activity or speech ceases. The child may stop talking in mid-sentence or cease walking. One to several seconds later, speech or activity resume. If standing or walking, a child seldom falls during one of these episodes.

"Spells" can be infrequent or very frequent, occurring many times per hour. Up to hundreds of seizures can occur in a single day. They may occur for weeks to months before they are noticed. They can interfere with school function and learning. Teachers may often interpret these seizures as lack of attention or other misbehavior.

No cause can usually be found for typical petit mal seizures. Anticonvulsant (anti-seizure) medications usually mitigate the symptoms quickly.

Source: National Institute of Health

http://www.nlm.nih.gov/medlineplus/ency/article/000696.htm

TIR with a Child Struggling with Complicated Grief and Diagnosed with ADHD and Clinical Depression

It is an exciting challenge to adapt approaches and tools to the child's constellation of abilities and problems. Given the repetitive nature of Traumatic Incident Reduction, it was instructive, therefore, to explore how a child identified as traumatized, clinically depressed and having Attention Deficit Hyperactivity Disorder would process trauma using TIR. This case report will present the experience of Scott, a 12-year-old when I first saw him.

Background

When first practicing TIR in 1997, I gingerly incorporated it into my existing practice. At that time, I mainly provided assessments and treatment to children from birth to their 19th birthday in a Children's Mental Health Unit at a local hospital in Ontario, Canada. After practicing TIR successfully for several years and applying it in as many situations as possible, I began to wonder how effective it would be for a child struggling with extreme difficulties of focus and attention.

He was the youngest of four and was in extreme distress. Scott's parents had separated five years previously, when he was age seven. His mother had just now recently begun to date and had strong feelings for the man she was dating. Scott and his siblings had met this man four months prior and now Scott was in complete distress. When not in tears, Scott was raging and sullen. He was in daily conflict with his mother and loudly accused her of not loving him anymore and of choosing her new partner over him. His mother was horrified by these accusations. The conflict with Scott further upset her as she and Scott had been very close over the years during his early history of medical problems. She felt guilty about Scott's enormous distress. She also felt angry that her decision to have a love partner after five years of devotion to meeting the needs of her children exclusively was met with such resistance. She badly wished for her cherished child to come to like and appreciate this fine man.

Scott's early life had been fraught with the fear that he would die. At age two, he was diagnosed with Childhood Leukemia. He immediately began a five-year regimen of treatment designed to save his life. The regimen included radiation of his brain, chemotherapy and other interventions.

The treatment was intensive and involved numerous injections. As a result he had a port inserted into his chest to receive medication. Throughout the five years, his blood was analyzed and there were numerous emergency trips to the hospital whenever he came into contact with a virus or a developed a slight fever. Given the absence of a strong immune system, what seemed like minor annoyances to a healthy child became potentially life threatening to him. His mother worried constantly that she would lose him and they became strongly bonded in the shared fear of loss.

Scott was fortunate in that the Leukemia went into remission and remained so. His five years of intensive treatment, and missed time at school and with friends, finally came to an end. His family could try to begin to build a more stable life. Unfortunately during this prolonged crisis-filled period, Scott's parents grew apart as they tried to meet the needs of their four children while his father worked at a demanding job. About six months following his successful treatment, Scott's father left the family. He bought a home nearby and made arrangements for his children and their mother to continue to live in their family home. Despite the mourning involved, his parents had organized a regular visiting schedule and communicated peaceably for the most part. In the intervening years, Scott's father had remarried and had another child. Scott and his siblings had the freedom to visit their father and stepmother and had adjusted well to these changes.

Need for Treatment

His mother's decision to enjoy a love relationship, however, threatened Scott's sense of security and evoked the terror of abandonment. Scott had yearly follow-up with the regional hospital in regard to his Leukemia. In the years following his treatment, he was diagnosed with ADHD and learning disabilities. It was Scott's understanding that the treatment designed to save his life had created some brain damage. It was not uncommon for children to later be diagnosed with anxiety disorders, ADHD and learning disabilities. He was offered medication to assist with the ADHD but declined to take them. This decision was supported by his parents. Scott did receive some assistance in the school system in response to his diagnoses. Given his presenting symptoms and inability to cope in any area of his life, Scott was seen by the clinic Psychiatrist who diagnosed him with clinical depression and started him on antidepressants.

Our shared plan was to assist Scott with a treatment approach to reduce his distress and to strengthen his coping. He would be safely weaned off the medication after a six month period of stability. Should any other issue arise, therapeutic support would be given to assist him to maintain his gains.

Impact of TIR

Scott was motivated to stabilize himself and gain relief from his anxiety, sadness and rage. He agreed to try TIR and was introduced to the approach through practicing the protocol on an innocuous time period of his life. After this, Scott's first TIR session lasted forty minutes. The incident he chose to work on was the day his father had told him of the separation, took his belongings, and drove away. Scott quickly oriented himself to this past event and was heavily abreactive. He vividly described his heartbreak over seeing his father driving away and his running after the car. He found it difficult to go through it each time, wondering aloud, and hoping each time that he was done. He stayed with it, however, until following the fourth run through when he announced that he was finished. Although surprised by the suddenness of this announcement, we ended the session even though I wondered about its effects.

Two weeks later, Scott's mother told me that significant settling had occurred: Scott had become less confrontational. Although he was not interested in spending time with his mother and her new partner, he was less rejecting. He was no longer experiencing outbursts and his anxiety appeared to be lower.

Scott related that he no longer had the image of his father driving away play in his mind. He talked about wanting to see his mother happy, but not being sure about this new person. The intensity of his fear of abandonment was gone and was replaced by wondering how he would fit with his mother and her new partner. He also began to talk about his need to spend time with his friends and his wish for his mother to understand this and not request his involvement in outings. This left the door open for some family sessions, focusing on Scott letting his mother know of his needs and negotiating appropriate closeness and distance relative to his age and stage of development.

His mother became aware of her own separation issues arising from Scott's push to involve himself more appropriately with peers. She completed her own TIR session on the theme of "Fear of losing Scott". One of the benefits of this work was his mother's recognition that she was pushing her children and her partner to connect rather than allowing for a natural process to occur. Recognizing the pressure she was bringing to the situation, she was then able to sit back and let those she loved come to know one another and find their own points of contact.

With less pressure to engage in a relationship with his mother's new partner, Scott began to interact more often and found shared areas of interest with this man. He was sincerely glad to see his mother happy. He also saw the efforts this man made to support her. As a result, he felt less threatened by this man's connection to his mother and less jealous of the time they spent alone.

Scott continued to make gains. Six months later, he pushed for a re-evaluation of his medications, and given his emotional stability, was assisted to withdraw from the anti-depressant.

Two months later, we were saying goodbye at the end of treatment. Scott was successfully managing himself and had strengthened his relationship with both parents. He also had begun to establish a friendly relationship with his mother's partner. He had come to realize and accept that this man could be in his life for many years to come. He could freely have a relationship with him without feeling disloyal to his father or fearing his father's abandonment of him.

Although Scott's ability to sustain attention was fleeting at times, he was able to successfully process the past events to an end point. His extreme distress promoted high motivation to stay with it, despite finding the repetition difficult. Scott found the sessions helpful but chose not to use TIR to address any other issue. His ability to finish the work on the incident he did complete, however, settled him and helped him to shift into more age-appropriate behaviors. Scott's rapid resolution of the first incident also demonstrated the variation that exists for individuals in coming to the end points necessary to resolve trauma.

	Trauma Resolution in an At–Risk
9	**Youth Program**
	By Teresa Descilo, MSW, CTS

Since 2001, Victim Services Center of Miami has received funding from the Department of Juvenile Justice in Florida to help at-risk youth resolve the impact of trauma. At-risk youth were defined as children who had risk factors in three of four domains: school, family, substance abuse and behavior. We first provided services at Madison Middle School, an inner city school in the Miami area zip code with the highest juvenile crime rate. Madison has approximately 1300 students from grades six to eight. In a recent year, 20.7% of the students missed more than a month of school per year. Compared to schools nationwide, Madison ranks below the 30th percentile in math and reading skills. One out of six students qualifies as learning disabled. A typical year sees about 300 incidents of crime and violence (see distribution in Fig. 9-1). The most common violation of the Student Code of Conduct at Madison is fighting. As one Assistant Principal explained, sixth graders are immature, "They look at each other = they fight." (CRP { Civil Rights Project}, 2000)

Simply outlawing violence in schools doesn't work. In reaction to nationwide outrage at highly publicized gun incidents, many school districts instituted a Zero Tolerance policy wherein any weapon infraction could result in a compulsory lengthy suspension or expulsion. Madison's principal, Thelma Davis, contributed to the controversial report, "Opportunities Suspended: The Devastating Consequences of Zero Tolerance and School Discipline" (CRP, 2000) which rebuts this approach. The report concludes:

> The increasing use of "zero tolerance" practices throughout the country is denying thousands of children opportunities for education, and alienating more from the educational process. Moreover, data clearly shows that minority students are frequently far more harshly disciplined than their white counterparts for similar, or less serious, offenses. Zero Tolerance is unfair, is contrary to the developmental needs of children, denies children educational opportunities, and often results in the criminalization of children.

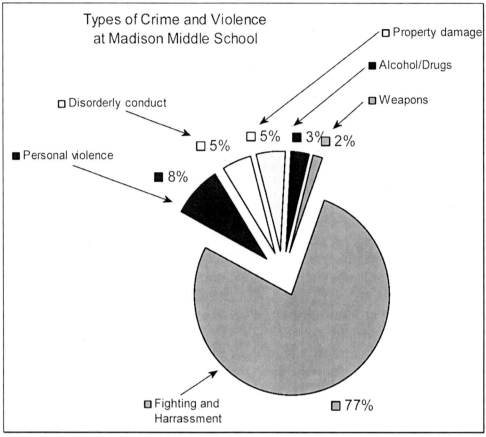

Fig. 9-1: Distribution of Crime and Violence at Madison
Source: www.schools-data.com

Victim Services of Miami was originally invited into the school by the school social worker in order to provide bereavement groups, because many children at the school lost caregivers to AIDS and homicide. Many of the children we served were from these bereavement groups. Others were from the severely emotionally disturbed group and many more were referred by the school social worker who had identified that they had overwhelming trauma in their lives.

Trauma and Childhood

Our understanding of trauma in children is strongly informed by the work of Ricky Greenwald, Ph.D. of Mt. Sinai Medical Center. In his book (Greenwald, 2002) he documents the role of trauma in conduct disorder, antisocial behavior and delinquency. This book also highlights the success of trauma-informed and competent services for at-risk youth.

Another influence in our thinking is Bruce Perry, M.D.'s research on child maltreatment. Perry explains how persisting fear can alter the developing child's brain. Specifically, these early traumatic events contribute to schizophrenia in patients who have a genetic predisposition. The neuron-developmental costs of adverse childhood events can no longer be ignored. In (Franey, Geffner & Falconer, 2001), Perry states that children with PTSD as a primary diagnosis are often labeled with Attention Deficit Disorder with Hyperactivity (ADHD), major depression, oppositional defiant disorder, conduct disorder, separation anxiety or specific phobia. Underlying this is the idea that the brain forms in a use-dependent fashion. Childhood is a critical and sensitive period for brain development; disruptions at these times may lead to abnormalities or deficits in neurodevelopment. Experiences of over-activation of important neural systems during sensitive periods of development can manifest in several ways, including:

- Maladaptive organization and compromised functioning in:
  - humor, empathy, attachment and affect regulation
  - being insensitive to any replacement experiences later in life, including therapy
- Being stuck in hyper-arousal or dissociation
  - males tend to manifest hyper-arousal
  - females tend to manifest dissociation
- Fear becomes a trait:
  - Very easily moved from mildly anxious to feeling threatened to being terrorized
  - Maladaptive emotional behavioral and cognitive problems arise

[Aggressiveness is often a reaction to chronic fear. – Ed.]

Treatment Approach

Traumatic Incident Reduction was our primary approach. The only difference in how it was delivered to children was that we incorporated some sort of craft activity that the children would engage in as they recounted their traumatic incidents. Beadwork turned out to be the most popular activity for both girls and boys. It seems that pairing a relaxing, right-brain activity with an initially distressing right brain activity lowered the arousal for the children through recounting rapes, beatings and homicides.

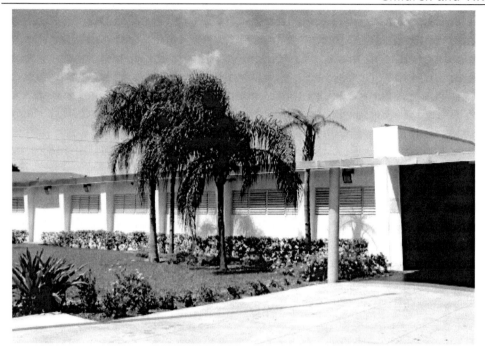

Fig. 9-2: Madison Middle School

The following data is for the 2003 academic year. Two factors limited our impact on the student body to thirty-five students during year three. Funding was the primary limiting factor and secondarily children had to have three out of four of the aforementioned domain risk factors [school, family, substance abuse and behavior]. It should be noted that the Madison Middle School program is strictly a pilot project, the purpose of which is to see what outcomes are possible, rather than a research driven project.

Measurement Scales Utilized

Our treatment approach used four different scales to pre- and post-test the children on the impacts of trauma on their lives.

- Child Report of Post-traumatic Symptoms (CROPS) (Greenwald and Rubin, 1999) – with a clinical cut-off of 19

- The Depression Self-Rating Scale (Birleson, 1981) – 13

- Self-Concept Scale for Children (Lipsitt, 1958)

- Youth Coping Index (McCubbin, Thomposn, and Elver) – acceptable range -91.8 to 95.4

Case Summaries

Two of the thirty-five cases are highlighted here in brief:

Case #1: A 12-year-old Hispanic female, she was a victim and witness of abuse, in the Florida Department of Children and Families system. She underwent 14 hours of individual treatment with TIR and 12 hours of group therapy over a seven month period:

Measurement	Pre-test	Post-test
Student Form	19	0
Depression SRS	15	0
Self-Concept Scale	88	109
Youth Coping Index	53	102

After treatment, she wrote:

> "The changes I've had ever since I started sessions here is I don't think I have to be perfect any more to impress my friends. Ever since I stopped trying to be perfect, my friends said I have become a better artist and a better friend. And I have become a better person as well."

Case #2: A 15-year-old African-American female, who was the victim of sexual abuse, who was a drug abuser and a runaway. Labeled as Oppositional Defiant, she underwent fifteen hours of individual treatment with TIR.

Measurement	Pre-test	Post-test
Student Form	39	6
Depression SRS	18	2
Self-Concept Scale	47	102
Youth Coping Index	71	128

After treatment, she wrote:

> "I know that my behavior changed: my attitude, my ways and also my language. And the service helped me a lot because I don't do bad things anymore or don't follow people. And my grades in school has improve a lot with As, Bs, Cs in conduct."

Results

First, I need to emphasize again that this was not a research project; the statistics gathered were in the interest of practicing responsibly. Children measured in the study all had symptoms of traumatic stress. Although there was no attempt to diagnose for PTSD, many of the children were above the PTSD cutoff on the Student Form and Depression Self-Rated Scale. Both scales show children significantly below the PTSD cutoff levels following treatment, as the following charts indicate:

Fig. 9-3: Average Results from Pre- and Post-Tests (N=35)

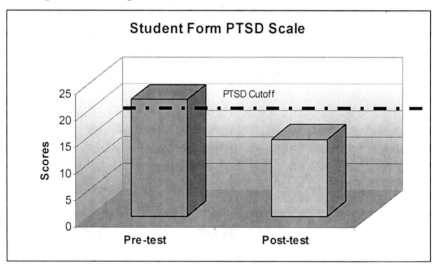

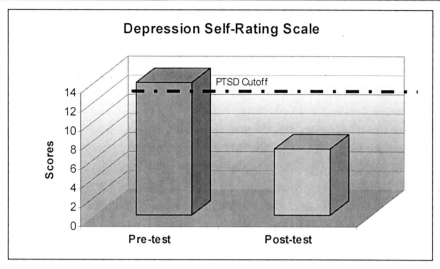

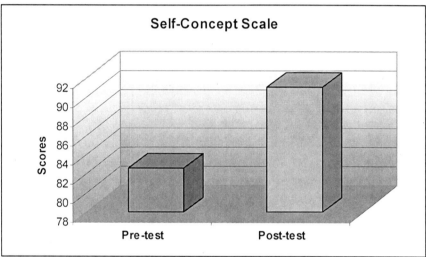

[Ed. Note: Average data for the Youth Coping Index was not available at time of going to press.]

Summary

We have heard from the school social worker at Madison Middle School that our trauma-focused program is the most effective service received by her students. She has reported to me that the children who went through our program are doing better academically, and behaving better at school and at home. I see that this program will offer a deeper solution to stopping the cycle of violence and helping youth move out of the category of "At Risk" and into truly resilient people.

As of 2006, Victim Services Miami has completed its work with Madison Middle School and has since moved to delivering services at Martin Luther King Leadership Academy. No data is yet published from work performed at this new venue.

References

Depression self rating scale [DSRD] (1981). Birleson P. IN: Corcoran K & Fischer J (2000). *Measures for clinical practice: A sourcebook. 3rd Ed.* (2vols.) NY, Free Pr. V.1, 535-536.

Self concept scale for children [SC] (1958). Lipsitt LP. IN: Corcoran K & Fischer J (2000*). Measures for clinical practice: A sourcebook. 3rd Ed.* (2vols.) NY, Free Pr. V.1, 617-618

Youth coping index [YCI] (1995). McCubbin HI; Thompson A; Elver K. IN: Corcoran K & Fischer J (2000). *Measures for clinical practice: A sourcebook. 3rd Ed.* (2vols.) NY, Free Pr. V.1, 628-631

Franey, K., Geffner, R., and Falconer, R., Ed. (2001). *The Cost of Child Maltreatment: Who Pays? We All Do.* Family Violence and Sexual Assault Institute, San Diego, CA.. http://www.fvsai.org

Greenwald, R. & Rubin, A. (1999). "Brief assessment of children's post-traumatic symptoms: Development and preliminary validation of parent and child scales". *Research on Social Work Practice, 9,* 61-75.

Greenwald, R. (2002) *Trauma and Juvenile Delinquency: Theory, Research, and Interventions.* Haworth Maltreatment and Trauma Press.

Civil Rights Project, The & Advancement Project (2000). "Opportunities Suspended: The Devastating Consequences of Zero Tolerance and School Discipline Policies." Delivered at National Summit on Zero Tolerance (2000). The Civil Rights Project, Harvard University. http://www.civilrightsproject.harvard.edu/research/discipline/opport _suspended.php

<table>
<tr><td>10</td><td>

TIR & Art Therapy:
A Case Study

By Anna Foley Clinical Director,
Moorside Trauma Service, England
</td></tr>
</table>

This case study is an example of my work, where I have successfully used the integration of TIR and trauma resolution art psychotherapy.

In this case (as with many others) where a child has been referred to me with a one-off [one time] traumatic incident, I ask the child to go through the incident, silently first in image form, drawing frame by frame. I ask, "What is the first thing you remember happening that day?" (in place of: 'Go to the start and tell me when you are there'). For children, this often has significance. It may not truly be the very beginning of the day, but it's what the child retrieves and brings forth that is usually indicative of important therapeutic material.

Once all the images are made, I then ask the child to go through the incident with the words "What happened?" As in pure TIR, I acknowledge each 'picture frame' and continue to elicit the event simply by saying 'What happened next?' or 'What happened after that?'

During this run-through, I ask particular questions about what they are viewing, trying to elicit each of the senses. This gives the child valuable time, and information about the impact of the event. It also provides both of us with information regarding any triggers. For instance I might say, "When you were lying on the floor, was there anything you could see, hear, smell?" etc.

In the third viewing I ask, "What were you thinking and feeling in this picture?" This allows a 'connecting up' of the facts, the senses and the thinking and feeling during and after the event.

About Matthew

Matthew was a Jamaican-English 14-year-old boy who was referred to me after an assault in which he was stabbed in the arm, and punched behind the ear, which causing swelling. Matthew was referred eight weeks after the incident.

Symptoms apparent upon referral:

- Withdrawal (leaving the house only with mother)
- Increased anger/aggression
- Hyper-vigilance

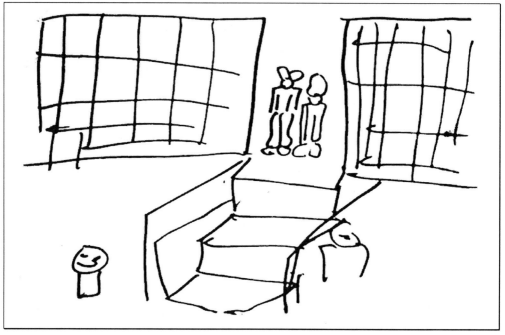

Fig. 10–1: Matthew's Picture #1

"What's the first thing you remember happening that day?" Matthew recalls going to the underground [subway] station with his friend, an ordinary day, having a laugh together. He doesn't remember anything particularly significant.

Matthew looks like he really has started with the beginning of the incident, so what was the significance of this first image of him and his friend? It transpired that Matthew's friend had run away (see picture 4), whilst the attackers pursued him, and this became a crucial part of Matthew's work with me: *trust of a friend.*

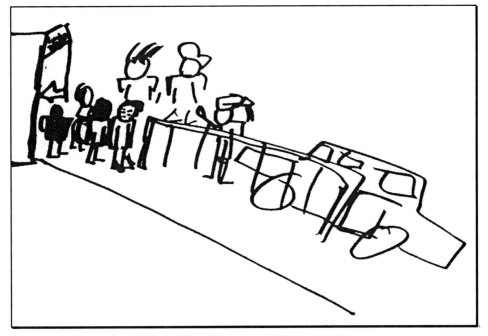

Fig. 10-2: Matthew's Picture #2

Matthew then recalls seeing a group of youths outside the station. There is some shouting going on, he's not sure what that was about. There is a person in the picture with a 'spotty face'.

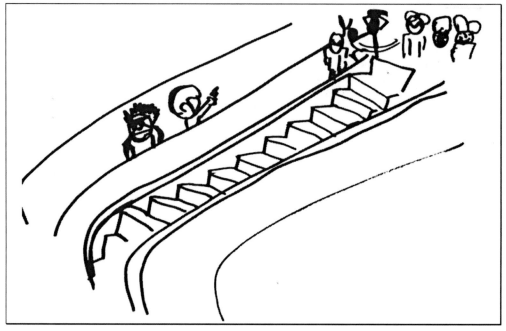

Fig. 10-3: Matthew's Picture #3

Matthew recalls going down the escalator with his friend, they appear to be being followed by the group of youths they'd seen outside the station. Matthew was not concerned, his friend however, was very anxious. It is his friend pointing to them in the picture.

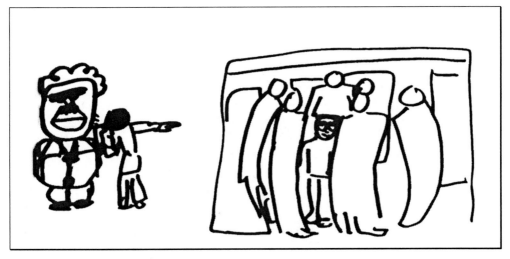

Fig. 10-4: Matthew's Picture #4

The group of youths surrounds Matthew in the train; he and his friend are separated. Matthew's friend told him he tried to get help (see left hand side of picture 4) Matthew doesn't believe him. Here the 'parallel stories' become obvious, and the therapeutic material becomes equal parts Matthew's experience of the assault, and the relationship issue with his friend.

Matthew describes here that he becomes frightened at this point but tries not to show it. He recalls seeing the boy with the spotty face. This kind of face was a trigger and something he was hyper-vigilant for if he was out with his mother.

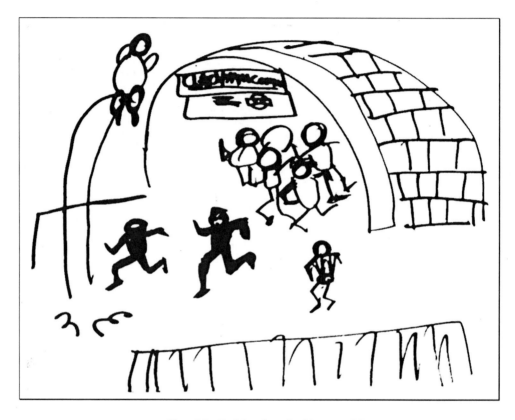

Fig. 10–5: Matthew's Picture #5

Matthew and his friend are chased out of the underground station. They are the two figures at the front. Matthew is cornered against some railings, his friend runs off (top left of picture). His friend tells him that he stayed and tried to fight the gang with him. Matthew recalls him running off and not being anywhere to be seen. Matthew recalls feeling helpless against this many people while on his own. He remembers deciding that he will 'take the beating'.

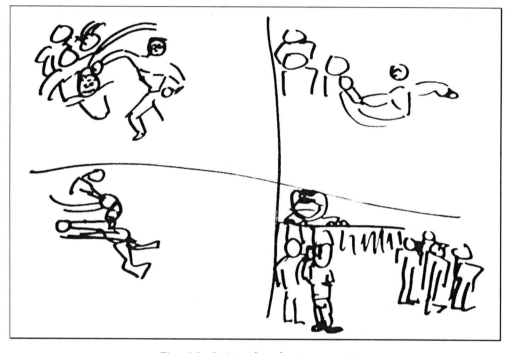

Fig. 10-6: Matthew's Picture #6

There are a lot of punches flying around. Matthew tries to fight back, but he is held by one of the gang whilst another punches him. Matthew finds it extraordinary that he can't really feel it. The pain doesn't come until later.

Matthew is stabbed by one of the gang in the left upper arm (see picture 7). The boy had a tracksuit on that said 'Tommy something' on it. Matthew was utterly shocked. He thought at first it was 'just a punch'. He remembers saying out loud "You stabbed me!" In retrospect he thought that sounded funny, but he had made the decision to 'take the beating', not imagining it would end up with a wounding and a scar for life. His friend is nowhere to be seen.

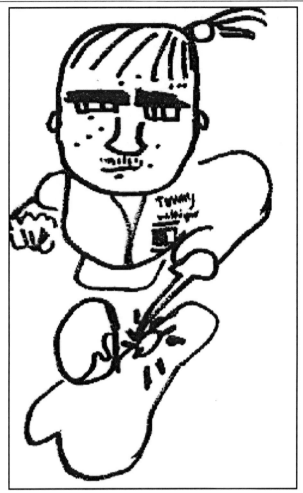

Fig. 10-7: Matthew's Picture #7

After the incident, Matthew was overwhelmed with anger, not because he had been stabbed but that he had been stabbed through his brand-new designer tracksuit. He remembers feeling through the hole in his tracksuit to the wound.

He is inconsolable when he realizes his friend had run away, and his friend might have been able to help him. (This of course may not have been the case, but the crucial part of it was that Matthew believed that was true, and now Matthew did not trust him).

What was more difficult for Matthew to accept was that his friend maintained he hadn't run away. Matthew felt angry, he felt his friend was lying, and he said he wanted his friend "To tell the truth."

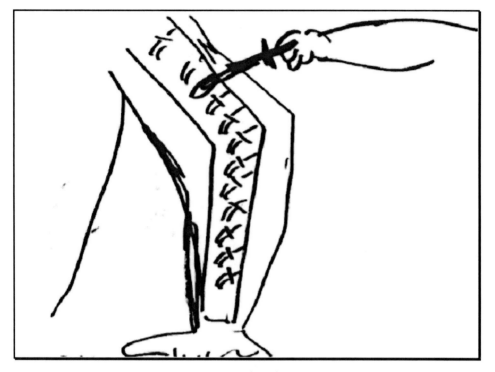

Fig. 10-8: Matthew's Picture #8

Pictures 9-11 show the wound as Matthew remembered it and its healing process. We did this after the incident was desensitized as a way of addressing his adapting and integration of having a lifelong scar. Matthew was able to conjure an image of the scar in the future, where it would be a little pink spot, with a memory attached.

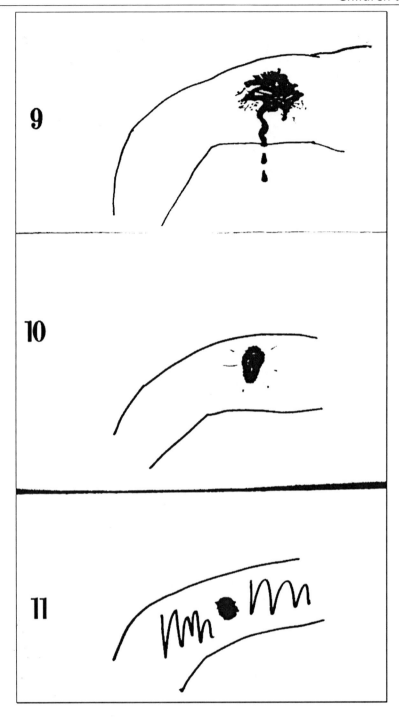

Summary

- Matthew's experience was fully desensitized.

- He regained his independence.

- He challenged his friend, and was able to work this out with him, and become good friends again.

- His hyper-vigilance subsided, but he became more street aware.

- His anger subsided upon the use of images to play out his revenge fantasies, and by sorting things out with his friend.

This treatment package lasted six sessions only. During follow-up with Matthew's mother some months later, it was reported that Matthew continued to be free of symptoms.

	# Anecdotal TIR Experiences with Children
	## Practitioner Interviews by Victor Volkman

In the interviews in this chapter, three experienced facilitators talk about their TIR work with children: Brian Grimes, Janet Buell and Alex Frater. Each brings a unique perspective to this use of TIR. Considered together, their observations provide a comprehensive overview of what you can expect to achieve using TIR and related techniques. – Victor Volkman

A Conversation with Brian Grimes

Victor: Tell me a little bit about your background.

Brian: I've been doing TIR and related techniques since the late 1980s and am currently a TIR Trainer in the Vancouver, BC area.

Victor: Do you find in general that the length of TIR sessions is different with children?

Brian: My experience has been that it's shorter. They tend to reach an end point more quickly. It seems to have something to do with the fact that they don't put a lot of added analysis or significance into the experience as adults often do.

Victor: It's more about, "What happened" as opposed to, "What it means that this happened to me?"

Brian: You got it exactly. They bleed off the emotion rather quickly, and they're done with it. They don't need to dissect it from any intellectual perspective.

Victor: Is this because they haven't built up a whole series of stories about how they were shaped by being a victim?

Brian: Yes, they don't have any fixed attitudes. It's just something that they had experienced. It was unfortunate or unpleasant, but that's what it was. They go through it and then they are done.

Victor: Are there any special techniques that you need to use to prepare children for TIR?

Brian: Sometimes I'll do some memory work with them to heighten their awareness of what it's like when they're in their mental environment.

Memory exercises help because they might have forgotten some of the content of their incident, or recalling it might be relevant to taking the charge off the episode. If I get them in there and I find that they're having a difficult time contacting the incidents, sometimes what we'll do is scale back and do a little more memory work and then go back to TIR work. *[See Appendix A for examples. – Ed.]*

Victor: Do you mean, for instance, recalling pleasant experiences?

Brian: Yes. I'll check what perceptions they are able to remember in recalling an earlier time, etc. Most children I've worked with just jump right into TIR though.

Victor: Do you find end points to be different with children?

Brian: Yes I do; the contrast would be that children report, "It feels better" or "It's OK now." Adults will tend to be more philosophic about how they viewed it vs. how they view it in the present (after doing TIR).

Victor: Some say that children often seem to lose interest in the incident or gain interest in something else. Do you find that true?

Brian: Yes, exactly. Their attention span is much, much shorter. Yeah, "That one's fine... Let's move on," or "What's next?"

Victor: Do you find you have to modify the language or the procedure to be less sophisticated with children?

Brian: No. I found the nomenclature, wording, and steps to be comfortable, but I make sure that I do a "practice run" with them before we actually get into anything. I go over the questions and directives so that they have the procedure clearly in mind. This allows me to open my mouth as little as possible and they know what I'm asking for and why. I'll say:

> "I'm going to create an incident here. What I want you to do is, when I say start, that's when I want your camera rolling. Very closely watch what it is that I do, every movement, every expression of my face, very closely. Then when I say stop, turn your camera off. Then what I'm going to do is walk you through exactly what happened and have you tell me what you saw."

I pick up a pencil or something from the desk, toss it in the air, catch it, and then give a puzzled look at the pencil, then I look at them, and say "stop." Then I walk them through that with the actual steps of TIR. From that, they have a comparative base and an understanding of what TIR is.

Victor: He or she will say, "You caught it?"

Brian: That's right. I'll ask, "Was there anything else you saw me do?" And the child will say, "No." I'll say, "Did you remember me looking at that pencil funny?" And then get, "Yeah, I did!"

Victor: That's interesting, because it also has the effect of bringing them into the present, if they were not quite there.

Brian: Exactly, because it takes them out of their head. They tend to enjoy it because it has a little bit of gamesmanship to it, which they like.

Victor: Is there some kind of minimum age or how would you decide whether or not to handle a particular child on the basis of maturity?

Brian: To be honest, I don't put an age limit on it all. If they are really young, I wouldn't follow the exact same series of steps. I would basically just do a very lightweight technique to try to get them to go through it and just tell me: What did you notice happened? How did you feel? I keep it kind of light but the principal thing is to get them to communicate. Get them to tell what is going on and what their perception is, and how they felt. If they're rather young, you really don't have them very long before they're bouncing all over the place wanting to do something else.

[Ed. Note: This is the Conversational Remedy, recommended for children and taught in the TIR Workshop.]

Victor: Are there any special challenges in working with children as opposed to adults?

Brian: Only the attention span. Sometimes what I've found is that if I work with a known incident [Basic TIR], where we have a known event that happened such as a bicycle accident where they were injured, I could do only what I could within the short time frame of that session, knowing full well that it hadn't been completely resolved. In other words, it still had bite to it. Then I come back and revisit it over a series of sessions until we get it to a proper end point.

Victor: Are there any particular types of incidents that are more prevalent with children as opposed to adults?

Brian: The incidents seem to be mostly about social interactions, as opposed to losses or accidents.

Victor: Are there any memorable cases you can share with me?

Brian: The strangest one I ever did was with the 8-year-old boy who was having nightmares that were getting more amplified and more disruptive. His dad thought it might be a good idea if I would work with the boy. I told the parent, "I'm happy to do it, but what we don't know is whether this child is going to be willing and how much we're going to be able to do."

I ended up interviewing the boy. The dreams had to do with fire. In my interview, I was asking a lot of questions: Have you been playing with matches? Were you burned recently? Were you playing with magnifying glasses? Did you see anything burning lately? None of these were the stimulus at all; I could tell he was being honest. He said, "It just suddenly started. I was watching Discovery Channel about the Apollo mission."

He didn't know about the Apollo 1 fire. The event that unfolded in the TIR session was what sounded like a replica of what might have happened if one had been present for that. I just let it go, but at first he was a little "weirded out" by it. He said "What is this?" I said "It's OK, it is whatever it is; just let it unfold and we'll keep going." He said "OK."

We just kept at it. His descriptions were rather interesting: a gloved hand reaching up and checking toggle switches, but he didn't have any basis of comparison for that. He heard chatter inside a helmet, clipped communications, checking items off, and then all hell broke loose. He was struggling to get out and couldn't. Here was a child not old enough to be alive when the event happened. It was the only session I ever gave him and the nightmares stopped. The session was just over an hour and 20 minutes and he returned to being a happy kid.

Victor: He not seen the documentary on the Apollo 1 fire?

Brian: No, what he had seen was the initial stages going into the Apollo program. They hadn't even gotten to that segment yet.

[As always in TIR work, no interpretation or evaluation is made of any material a client comes up with. Experience and results have reinforced our adherence to this axiom. –Ed.]

Victor: Are there any other client stories you can share?

Brian: There was a boy who had been hit by a motorcycle and there was a really severe wound that went all the way to the femur bone. I took him actually out to the accident site and walked him through it and had him show me where it happened, what his body position was, and then we did TIR on it. The pain turned on in the femur pretty strongly in the course of the session. He was fascinated by that.

Victor: How did it change through various viewings? Did it become more intense, or less?

Brian: There was no pain at all when he first made contact with the incident. Then on subsequent times through, the pain intensified and actually got pretty severe. He wanted to discontinue at that point. I let him know that that was normal and if we were to just continue then we would get through it. Fortunately, we stayed with it and it did resolve. He was pretty happy with that.

[While the rules that structure and govern this work are clear that a client is never forced, or asked to do more than he or she can do, at times, with encouragement, a client will be able to continue through something difficult and reach a resolution. Clients often feel quite triumphant at having gotten through something that they thought they might not be able to do. –Ed.]

Victor: Afterwards his symptoms were considerably less?

Brian: You bet, yes. I spoke with his mom and she said ever since that session the healing process just seemed to go so much faster. He talked about what had happened without emotion but more matter-of-factly, as something that just happened. I've done many, many sessions and very few caused a reliving of the pain, certainly not this intense.

Victor: Do you find that there's any relationship with trauma and dyslexia?

Brian: Yes, on an emotional level, you bet. My theory is that we're recording everything that happens, whether we like it or not. So those memories are locked up and if there's a humiliating experience that was emotionally traumatic and you get the person anywhere near similar circumstances to what existed back then, they can trigger right back into it. There were a few times, not many, but there were a few times where I actually had to use TIR working with people doing the dyslexia program.

Victor: Because they got restimulated [triggered]?

Brian: Yes, they were right there in the memory. The counselor would just say, "I have no idea what to do with this. The student tells me about it but is not getting calmer, but getting more upset." I would just take over and do a TIR session. It would be pretty fast usually. There's definitely a use for TIR in dealing with study problems.

A Conversation with Janet Buell

Janet Buell has received a BA in Education and is an ordained minister. She is a member of the International Pastoral Association, an ecumenical group of pastoral counselors. She is the author of more than a dozen books including *Emotional First Aid*. Janet has been a TIR facilitator for many years.

[Conversational TIR, often used with children, is taught in the TIR Workshop, Level One. The other sorts of remedies Janet refers to are taught on the second level TIR workshops; see Appendix B - Ed.]

Victor: Tell me about some of the outstanding experiences you've had working with children.

Janet: One that comes to mind is a 12-year-old girl I worked with. This is a child of color who had lost both parents. I took a while assessing her to see how mature she was. First, I checked to see if she would be able to sit still through the procedure and secondly to find out how good her ability to recall things was to see if she was a candidate for TIR. When I first saw her, she appeared much more mature than the average kid of that age. I started the procedure as usual and she actually spent several hours on it. It was a somewhat shocking and unexpected loss for her, an automobile accident. She did very well with it.

She spotted the moment when she'd first heard that it had occurred, and some of the decisions she'd made. One was never to be a parent herself, because if you were never a parent then you could never cause that kind of loss for someone else. That was the decision that had the potential to impact her life most heavily. It was about three months after the accident occurred when I worked with her. She did, quite naturally, after reducing some of the charge from the incident, realize that it had also been extremely upsetting when her grandmother had passed away. The incident had been similar in the sense that it was also a shock to her. I probably would not have pursued it because she had expressed a realization, but she seemed to have a lot of energy left. She seemed OK, so I sent her back and had her tell me about the loss of her grandmother.

That incident was much lighter in the sense that it didn't take nearly as much time as her parents' loss. She realized that the prior loss of her grandmother had actually lightened the shock when her parents died because she had already found out that you might lose someone suddenly. She realized that she had sort of distanced herself. The reason she had seemed so old and wise for her age was because she had realized with the earlier loss at age seven or eight that you couldn't always depend on someone to be there. Her words were, "It was almost like I started preparing to lose mommy and daddy because I already knew that something like that could happen." She did have some realizations then about the way that that had altered her behavior to have had the loss of her grandmother happen early in her life.

I remember her making some observations about other children having a little different attitude about life. She related good and bad things; that she always feared another major loss and that caused her to be more fearful in general. She also realized that it had made her more mature than other kids her age. So she felt that the earlier loss had mixed outcomes. In some ways it was a blessing because she mentioned that she had always been very certain of the importance of maintaining communication with her parents and not holding onto any upsets with them. I believe that with her grandmother there had been a little bit of an upset with her before she passed away and the girl vowed not to let that happen again. She was always very careful to make sure that if she and her parents were going to be separated, that they were on very good terms. Her overall realization was that at least she had succeeded in not having any upsets between herself and her parents when they died. Also that she always made a point that if they were going to be separated for any length of time to make sure that she told them she loved them. Those are the nature of the realizations that she gave me.

Victor: Did she have any classic trauma symptoms like nightmares and intrusive thoughts?

Janet: Her aunt was the person who'd brought her to me. The girl was being very brave about it but she was very concerned any time her aunt went anywhere. She was having nightmares and her biggest concern was much too strong a fear that she would continue to lose other people. She was very a serious girl. If her aunt was going out to get the mail, she felt she had to tell her she loved her. Her aunt was the one who took over her care after her parents died. It got to the point where her aunt felt that the girl couldn't go through her life focused on that. It was an extreme fearfulness of losing someone. That was the prime manifestation. Fortunately, she got her to me fairly soon after the accident. I think it came up when she didn't want to go to a school event that would have required her being away from her aunt. It seemed as though her fear of being separated was too strong for her to have fun on this trip. That was the presenting reason that her aunt saw that it could be real trouble for her in the future.

Victor: You've got a really good memory for detail, thank you for that story.

Janet: She was an extraordinary child. I've probably done several thousand hours of TIR, but this one made quite an impact on me.

Victor: Let's talk about how you modify things for younger children. Can you give me some specifics?

Janet: When I have a young child who has had a loss, I spend quite a bit more time doing remedy type things in terms of focusing attention on the environment. I work in shorter sessions and use a somewhat less formal procedure, watching more closely for signs of tiredness. I would probably also focus on having the child look at one particular portion of what occurred rather than the whole incident on the first round. I simplify the terminology.

Victor: By portion, do you mean addressing one part or aspect of the incident?

Janet: It would depend a lot on what the incident was. With children, I watch much more closely for signs of fatigue and signs of their attention going off the incident. I may settle for their talking about one aspect of a traumatic incident and brightening up some. I know that there might be more work needed on it, but I do it over several sessions so that the attention span isn't as big a factor. A lot depends on their engagement; if they get into it I certainly won't leave them. I stop at a point of relief even if I wasn't necessarily convinced that it was over. I might then choose to take it up again on another day if there were still interest and attention tied up in the incident.

Ordinarily, if I'm working with adults, I schedule as much time as needed and try to get them through to a full end point in one session. But a child might not have the attention span or the stamina for that. On the other hand, I've had a few small children who were so fixated on an incident that there wasn't anything else they could pay attention to. It probably depends on the degree of the trauma.

Victor: I think I've heard that from a few practitioners that they may spread the incident out over three or four separate sessions.

Janet: I think it depends. If the child is completely fixated on it and stuck on it then you might as well feed them well, get them well rested, and do as much as you can to prepare for a longer session. But if it's something that affects the child only sometimes and they are not totally fixated on it, then I would probably try to do some lighter remedies rather than go into TIR right away.

Victor: Are there any other cases that stand out in your memory?

Janet: I worked with an interesting boy who was sixteen at the time but seemed much younger. I believe the official diagnosis for him was "mild autism". Even though he was sixteen or seventeen, he acted more like a child of about nine or ten. He had suffered a loss; he had been attending a residential school that had been helping him a great deal. I don't remember the exact circumstances, perhaps the school had closed but there was a reason he could no longer live there. He had quite a loss from that. The parents were trying to find an alternative place for him to get the kind of care he needed. He was very fixated on the friends he no longer saw, and even more on the resources which the school had provided. He was very upset and seemed incapable of understanding that they didn't have a choice in the matter. He was upset with his parents and upset with the school.

I worked with him as though he were more like eight or ten years old and did more of a Conversational TIR remedy with him. It stood out in my mind because it did go well. He didn't necessarily have the usual things you look for in an end point, and I had to go more by the fact that by one point his parents took him to visit another facility that might be able to keep him there and he seemed interested. It was the fifth or sixth place they looked at, but it was no better or worse than those they had already seen. I did work with him over the course of several sessions.

Victor: Rather than dramatic realizations, he just got to a point of acceptance?

Janet: Yes, he talked to me a great deal about the place he'd been that was so important to him. He was very focused on counting. He was a child who could tell you the ZIP code [postal code] or area code of any place in the world. So it was a loss of things that he had used. It was a very unusual situation but they were very real losses, including some kind of computer program that he was interested in developing. He was apparently quite good at it and he was worried about being able to use his strengths at another school. Even though he had been to other schools that could provide that could provide similar services, he wasn't ready to accept that. When they took him to the last one, they felt like he was finished working with me because he was ready to go to that school.

I had to view it his way and see what a big loss it had been for him. Some things might be hard for an average person to understand, such as how he would miss this one project he was working on. I heard from his parents that he did very well at the new facility. It's kind of a case where you realize that someone with a mental illness can be traumatized just like the rest of us. The end point is not necessarily that they are going to be cured of that mental illness, it's just that they have dealt with the loss. So you have to change your standards. I didn't think that it was going to cure autism, and it didn't, but it made him a happier autistic kid.

Victor: I've heard the same thing with regards to dyslexia. You can develop incidents around dyslexia.

Janet: That's true actually. I've dealt with quite a few people on the subject of dyslexia in regaining their self-confidence because that was lost as a result of how they were treated more than from the dyslexia. I've actually treated a few young people with that.

A Conversation with Alex Frater

Alex D. Frater is a psychotherapist, Certified Forensic Trauma Specialist, and clinical hypno-therapist. He has been practicing in Campbelltown, Australia since 1986. Originally schooled in Rational Emotive Behavior Therapy (REBT), he now uses Traumatic Incident Reduction (TIR) and Applied Metapsychology techniques a great deal. I spoke with Alex about how he uses TIR in several aspects of his private practice.

Victor: What was your practice like prior to learning TIR and how did it change?

Alex: By the early 1990s, my workload had consistently reached 70 hours a week (Monday – Friday, 8 am to 10 pm) and had started to encroach on my weekend. I found that some of my patients would get better using REBT, and while it helped a lot of patients, some it didn't. I started looking around the world for different ways of handling trauma. I read Robert Moore's paper[1] and spoke with him and that inspired me to get TIR training in the USA.

The whole idea behind learning TIR was hopefully to: (1) decrease my workload and, (2) to be more efficient with my patients. I became much more efficient with my patients, but it did nothing for my workload. Being more efficient meant that I was getting more referrals. In the area here, probably 18-20 medical practitioners use me and 85% of my practice is medically referred. In the early stages, the local psychiatrist had used me quite extensively. I nearly always had five or six of his patients in my practice. I found TIR certainly much more efficient, but it was my fault that I wanted to reduce my workload and I did nothing about that. I think I can say that anybody whom I used TIR on for various traumas was successful. It's certainly extremely valuable in making me more efficient and it keeps my practice rolling along very, very well.

Because I've been trained in REBT (which is cognitive), I spend the first session doing a complete assessment. The second session, I spend an hour showing the concepts of REBT. I spend two or three sessions on that and give them handouts. When I first came back from my training, I started to do TIR straight off. I found that I got better results if I

---

[1] "Primary Resolution of the Post-Traumatic Stress Disorder"
http://www.tir.org/metapsy/moore_ret.htm

put it off a bit and did some basic work. That's seems to help people a lot.

Victor: Do you use TIR with children?

Alex: I do use TIR with children and they do run shorter sessions. I'm always amazed how quickly they can do it. One case that comes to mind is of a family where an eighteen month old baby slipped under the wheel of a 4-wheel drive truck that was backing up. It was a horrific accident; the child was killed as the vehicle ran over his head. There were four children in the family: a girl of ten, a boy of seven, another boy four years old, and the baby. The eldest child couldn't go near car parks [parking lots] after this incident. She was having flashbacks. We got her trauma resolved in about four sessions. I find that kids' ability to recover from trauma is incredible, absolutely incredible.

Another case I had a little while ago was a 12-year-old boy who had to sleep in his parents' bedroom the past four years. He was frightened to go to into his own bed and that sort of thing. I said to him, "When you go to bed, what happens in your mind? What kind of pictures do you have?" He said, "I'm just scared." I said, "I want to know the picture you see." He said, "People rob the place."

When I went to do TIR with him, he remembered that four years before, he'd heard a car stop at the front and doors banging. In his mind, he thought they were robbers. As time went on in his mind (none of this had happened) he imagined those people coming into the house, breaking the door open, and shooting his mother, father and sister. They point the gun at him and they are about to shoot him in the head. He was dreaming this too after awhile. None of this was true, but he had thought about it so much that it had become reality to him. We fixed him in three visits, just by running that scenario in his mind.

Victor: You, in essence, addressed the fantasy of the incident?

Alex: Yes. Before TIR, when he went to bed, he'd run that fantasy through his mind. He of course had all the emotions that went with it and he couldn't get it out of his mind until we used TIR on it.

Victor: Do you find end points different with children?

Alex: Yes, they are probably less dramatic. Mind you, I find some adults not very dramatic either. You have to be very careful with kids because they reach the end point sometimes quite quickly. I ask them, "How did it feel?" and they say, "Oh it feels quite good." But they don't go into raptures. I modify the language to be less sophisticated and I do that with adults too sometimes. I get doctors, lawyers, businessmen and I get some people who have barely borderline IQs. I change the language a little bit, but the handouts I give them are all at an adolescent reading level. Everybody gets the same handouts. I find some of the kids are pretty bright, and they handle it all right.

Victor: Any special challenges to working with children?

Alex: I find that they are a delight to work with. The sessions are generally not as long for a child as with adults. I've always booked longer hours with kids, but I've never ever needed it. I find usually 40 to 50 minutes is about as long as you want.

Victor: Some facilitators have told me that in working with children they need to spread out the incident over 2 or 3 sessions, only addressing part of it in each session. Do you find that to be the case?

Alex: You've got to watch because they get bored with it. When I notice that happening, I ask, "Do you feel OK?" They say, "Yeah, I feel good." So I say, "All right if we leave it here today?" On the other hand, often I've had no trouble with them covering the whole incident in a single span of time. That young girl with her brother being killed was able to go through the whole thing from the word go, up to and including the funeral she went to. The first session ran for an hour and twenty minutes.

In doing this, I find that the first time is a bit straggly. It's something that they've never seen done and they find it a bit weird I think. I don't worry unduly about the first one. It's mainly to get them going and using it. I find that the second session runs better; they don't find it strange. When I'm explaining it to them, sometimes I'll say, "It's a bit weird, isn't it? Most sessions we do comfortably within an hour, quite easily. If it's too long, they lose their power of concentration.

12 Parents' Success with TIR

Please see Chapter Six for notes on the subject of parents working with their children. The two very personal and moving stories in this brief chapter are told by parents who are not only excellent facilitators, but who are able to keep the objectivity and focus needed to work with their own children.

TIR and Early Childhood Trauma

By Tony DeMaria

I would like to share with you this anecdote of my son Tom's very early traumas, how they became restimulated/triggered many years later, and their successful resolution. The following article describes the scenario as it unfolded when Tom was age nine.

Tom and I have had some very basic Applied Metapsychology sessions pretty much every week for quite a while. On this occasion, I had just come home from a business trip to find my son unusually upset about a scene he saw in a recent children's movie, "Chicken Little." I recall that he walked up to me in a rather glum mood. He said that something in a movie made him sad and he wanted to have a session.

He asked me for a session and we went straight to it. At first we talked for a while about the movie. Then we explored his thoughts concerning the particular scene where Chicken Little thought the sky was falling and how it made him sad. We decided to use TIR. We had used Unblocking (See the glossary and the page after it), and grounding techniques many times in past sessions. However, this was Tom's first exposure to TIR.

The first few passes through the incident relieved him a bit, but left him with a sense of mystery. So, I asked him for an earlier similar incident. It was as if a storm had burst through the room. He was grieving in rhythmic heaves and barely able to articulate his words. When he was finally able to speak, he worked out the location of the incident. It had happened when he was two weeks old and was being taken away in an ambulance. The fear, thoughts and perceptions were coming apart in wave after wave of tears. It is times like these that you realize the importance of the Communication Exercises! (See glossary)

Some of the interesting highlights of his viewing were: the intense frustration and fear of not being able to communicate to the emergency medical technicians in the ambulance, his awareness of his parents in the car behind him, and him having no idea why this was happening. Much could be written concerning his perceptions as a two-week-old, not to mention his ability to recall it years later. Of course, the most important aspect was the fact he was confronting the most traumatic event in his short life and simultaneously releasing a massive amount of emotional charge about it.

As we made passes through the ambulance incident, he developed an ability to put aside parts of the incident that held no interest and continued to release charge from what was left. When we finally got toward the end, he was having fun with it; he eventually looked around and yelled, "I made it!" This sudden awareness that he had made it through all the trauma of his early life seemed to dissolve the last bit of charge for him. We ended the session and Tom went back to his room to play video games.

One of the residual effects of his early experiences was a primal terror that his parents had left him when they were not in view. This would cause him to run through the house crying and yelling. After the TIR session, this dissolved. He still wanted to know where we were, but he had dropped the blood-curdling screams and frantic behavior. His confidence in himself had changed dramatically. Although we were amazed at the change, Tom didn't seem to take any notice. He was content to know the sky wasn't falling after all.

Obviously, Tom has led an exceptional life. He is being raised in a non-violent and loving family. Nevertheless, he was born with a major congenital heart defect. He has received three open-heart surgeries with the last one being a miraculous repair, which is a story in itself. His surgeries were at two weeks, three years, and five years old. One of the interesting factors in childhood trauma is: what is considered trauma to the client? The actual surgeries have had no interest for Tom in terms of residual trauma. The key factors that have been addressed are: being left alone, being confined, and not knowing what is happening to him. Because we have found that his lack of knowing what was happening was a major source of upset, we have always made it mandatory that the doctors explain everything to him. This knowledge of what, how and why probably accounts for his ability to maintain a sense of safety and control during these risky procedures with minimal aftereffects.

Relieving Stuttering in a Young Child:

An Anecdote

Facilitator name withheld by request

How young can a child be and still do TIR?

Our son, Charlie, was two years old, and had recently learned to talk. He loved to communicate, and practiced at every opportunity. One day he started stuttering, not badly, but noticeably. It became worse, and within a few days he literally could not talk. We took him to the doctor and asked "What is wrong?"

"Don't worry," the pediatrician replied. "It's not unusual for children to stutter at this age."

"When will it get better?" we asked.

"Maybe in six months. Sometimes it takes years."

My husband and I looked at each other. Our son was already terribly upset, terribly frustrated. We knew he would never recover from such an inhibition of his ability to communicate.

We went home and we talked; we tried to figure out what might have caused this. It had started suddenly. Could something have triggered the stuttering? Then my husband remembered: a week earlier he and our son had gone out back of the day care center to look at large construction machines: tractors, backhoes, and such. Charlie had been fascinated, and father and son had a wonderful time looking at, touching, and talking about these amazing machines. The following day he had started stuttering. Could the machines have been a trigger?

Fools rush in where angels fear to tread. I didn't know that children as young as two couldn't be expected to use techniques such as TIR successfully. We were desperate and I was willing to try anything. After lunch, I sat down with Charlie and said, "Do you remember when you and Dad went to look at the big machines?" He said "Y-Y-yeah, b-i-ggggg m-m-m-achines".

"Tell me what happened."

He tried; he did his best to tell me. After a few minutes the terrible stuttering eased just a little.

[*Ed. Note: It is vital not to push a child past any kind of end point as that will cause the child to be unwilling to participate in the future. This facilitator is particularly adept at noting end points in children.*]

The next day I asked again. "Do you remember when you and Dad went to look at the big machines?" He nodded. "Tell me what happened." We went through the incident a few times, but there didn't seem to be much there.

What do you do when you've been through something and there's nothing more there? As far as I knew, this was the first time Charlie had seen such big machines since he was born.

I took a deep breath and asked, "Was there an earlier time when you saw the big machines?" Charlie looked at me and his attention went "zap" onto something. He started shaking and stuttering and nodding, and then he started laughing. He laughed for three or four minutes, and I laughed with him. He finally stopped and hiccupped, and we smiled at each other.

He never stuttered again.

13 TIR in a Mental Health Clinic Setting

Patricia Furze, MSW, RSW

Interviewed by Victor Volkman

Victor: Tell me a little bit about your background and work experience.

Patricia: After I completed my Bachelors of Social Work, I worked for the Children's Aid Society in Ontario. I worked there for a couple years and had an amazing experience with practice with families. It was a generalist position, so it allowed me to do a variety of interesting work. This was a child protection agency so our mandate was child protection and safety. As a generalist I was involved in protection investigations, placement of children in foster homes, group homes and residential care, adoption work and strengthening families through the provision of parenting groups, individual and family counseling. It was a resource-poor area so we also had the opportunity to create new programs. I was involved in creating a play therapy program with a family therapist and a professor from a nearby university. The tragedy in the lives of those children and parents and their resilience propelled me to pursue the goal of becoming a therapist who could assist people in transforming life's challenges into meaningful lives.

I returned to school and completed my Masters degree specializing in children and families. After graduation, I stayed in Toronto, Ontario and began working for a Children's Mental Health agency for the next ten years. I was intensively involved with street kids for about eight years and developed a model for working with them. We provided various therapies to address their mental health needs and develop skills. The goal was to assist them to sustain employment and manage relationships. This highly traumatized population taught me that trauma is replicated throughout the various systems that an individual engages with. As a result, we intervened to create and support healthy contexts with these youths to create meaningful change. It was an amazing period of growth for me in terms of understanding trauma and the basic needs that unite us as people in general. I also did consultations in our two residential programs. These care for adolescents, between ages thirteen to nineteen, with emotional and severe behavioral problems.

In the mid-1990s, I went to work at Markham Stouffville Hospital. They were opening a child and family clinic in mental health. They needed a team of people to actually develop the program and I was fortunate to be involved in the creation of it. It's a small community hospital that has a philosophy of empowerment for the frontline staff. Basically the unit was self-operating with the support of management. It has been a really exciting place to work and a wonderful clinic.

The team consists of a part-time psychiatrist, child psychologist, and two and half positions for social work. It's a really small clinic but it does amazing work. Over the past five years I've worked with my colleagues in creating a model that incorporates TIR. We've used TIR to assist when people were blocked by trauma, whether they were aware or unaware of what was blocking them, in order to get them past those blocks to support the child.

Victor: Can you take me through the steps that a patient entering the hospital would go through and how TIR works with the total treatment plan?

Patricia: Ours is an outpatient mental health clinic in a community hospital in a rapidly growing area north of the city of Toronto. The referrals are all from doctors who have a connection with the hospital. The doctors make the initial referral of the client, often with a question about severe behavioral problems or possible mental health concerns that need identification and treatment. It could be disruptive disorders, anxiety disorders, depression, or Post-Traumatic Stress Disorder. It's usually quite serious and often with children who have been suffering for some time. The physician offers support in the ongoing care over time and connects with this clinic to request assessment and treatment to address the presenting problem. We serve children from toddler-hood all the way up to their nineteenth birthday.

The referral is by phone and usually sent to the social work staff for assessment. The social work staff connects with the family and child during an office interview and assesses what the needs are at that time. The child psychologist may also attend initial screenings.

If she's running a particular depression group for example, she might screen for that particular depression group and assess needs. At that point, the person who assessed the family starts working with them, which allows for continuity of care. If it was determined at the time of assessment or afterwards that the child needed to be assessed by psychologists regarding diagnosis of anxiety, PTSD, or disruptive disorder then a referral would be made to the psychologist.

The other possibility is a need for psychiatric assessment in order for there to be some medication or diagnosis. There is a lot of interaction between the therapists and mental health professionals in order to support the individuals there for help.

The Child Part of a Family System

Primarily, the people identifying the need for TIR in a clinic are the social workers. For example, they may decide that a person could benefit from individual therapy and family therapy. They may work for some time with him/her trying to address the presenting issues with Cognitive Behavioral Therapy. They may find in that work that despite their best intentions and the hard work of the family, they are running into certain blocks which the individual isn't able to get past. Or they may find that they are able to resolve some things but they aren't able to maintain that level of resolution of the presenting problems over time. As well, we experience parents or children who don't seem able to integrate new skills despite their understanding and commitment to make changes.

The social workers flag those particular patients and speak to me (since I provide TIR for the group). We talk about the possibility of offering TIR and presenting it to the family and the individual involved. We talk to the family about what was happening and try to help them identify where the "stuckness" was associated in their life and find other times where they might have felt similarly. As a result, often the children, youth and/or parents became aware of something that may have happened in the past that was operating in the present without their being conscious of it. Through that recognition, they were often interested in doing a piece of work to resolve that stuck point in order to make progress again and gain relief from the problematic behaviors. Most of the time people are very interested in feeling better and gaining relief from what was happening. If this doesn't happen, they're very frustrated by their lack of progress. So offering TIR at this time is often really supportive. Initially they often feel ambivalent and wary because it's hard to confront difficult issues. But usually they are very much more interested in seeing what they can do support their child. This was one way the need for TIR was identified and offered.

[Sometimes the most important thing parents can do to help their children is to do their own trauma work. – Ed.]

Alternatively, at the intake level it will be noted that someone has had a trauma that seems to underlie the presenting problem. For example, someone could identify a loss and be experiencing complicated grief and therefore unable to get past the loss. Some individuals will tip you off by saying "a part of me died that day" or "I just haven't been myself since that person died" or "I haven't been able to even think about that person." Another typical scenario is a parent with a child who had a very serious childhood illness such as leukemia or another hard to diagnose illness. The child got hospitalized; the parents were really scared and didn't know what they are dealing with for a long time. It created a trauma for that family and then life carried on. The disease was identified and the child received treatment, but what lingered was the impact of that initial period of prolonged uncertainty and the fear that the child might die. These experiences could have been part of what is identified in the family's history. What currently is going on seems to replicate the fear of loss and feeling overwhelmed and anxious. We often see that in trauma, as it gets shows up in all kinds of different ways. So my colleagues, who were able to identify these patterns and the underlying trauma that was operating in the present, would refer to me to provide TIR on the unresolved trauma.

Once the TIR work was completed, the initial therapist again picked up the case. Often after the TIR work was completed, the family were interested in doing work on maintaining good and healthy boundaries, social skills, life skills, parenting skills and coping strategies. Once the charge from the underlying trauma had been released, parents and children were able to integrate new skills into their repertoire. This dynamic is really important for organizations to understand, as those individuals cost programs significantly in time and resources, as the unresolved trauma can block the integration of new learning. As well, the "stuckness" for the individual can be demoralizing, frustrating and create hopelessness. Family members can blame one another for the lack of progress, leading to further relationship breakdown.

Over the years, I have encountered many people who were offered all kinds of skill-building cognitive therapies to intervene in their patterns in a particular way, and who were unable to sustain growth despite cognitively understanding it, being very motivated, and able to understand their own patterns. They couldn't seem to maintain the growth that they were experiencing. Yet, often after TIR it would cease to be a problem. If someone had had a lot of work prior to TIR in terms of skill-building, it was likely to come together in a very different way following the TIR process and they would be bolstered by that earlier work. So, whether it came before or after, the skill-building could be integrated better after TIR had been completed. It seems that people's amnesic barriers become dissolved and it allows them more fluid access to their internal resources and as a result more stability emotionally. It's very exciting. I believe that adding the TIR approach to an existing clinic helps to shorten treatment time and costs and strengthens effectiveness and relief for individuals. It can help to address the "revolving door" that can plague mental health organizations.

Victor: Part of the Metapsychology theory is that when you release the traumas you have more free attention to do the things you want to do.

Patricia: Yes. In fact, we use that theory to educate the clients. That's one of the things I talk about with people around the benefits of pursuing TIR. One of the ways we did it was through identifying the parenting styles. Often we were dealing with families where the parents were traumatized and the kids were traumatized or where parents were traumatized and the kids were secondarily traumatized by the parenting style used. The parenting approach of a traumatized person can be very extreme: it can be either overly close or overly distant. It becomes very difficult for that parent to be consistent and to be able to be close to the child while holding them accountable. They get overly close to the child and over-identify and, therefore, not be able to hold them accountable and/or they get so angry and distant that they become harsh and ineffective in that approach.

Sometimes we talk about holding the children accountable in a loving way and helping parents to identify the stuck points around that experience. Other times we talk about the impact of the child's trauma on that parent's parental behaviors. For example, childhood leukemia treatment takes five years and can result in secondary trauma for the parent. So we look in both areas where the parent's history can impact the child and the child's history can impact the parent. Often we also see a situation where the child had an accident that a parent witnessed, and, therefore they had their own secondary trauma around it.

Trauma often compels us to act in a certain way, often unconsciously. If we made that understood, we found that people were more interested in doing the work. Also what excited them was the potential to do a chunk of work in a one-session format which allowed them to have resolution inside the single session. This was absolutely why people were more interested in TIR rather than pursuing a series of other interventions. They were more able to see themselves completing a chunk of work at once rather than attending sessions repetitively.

Victor: What kind of advice would you have for someone establishing a program like yours in a hospital or similar setting?

Patricia: I would definitely support them getting training in TIR and really understanding and practicing it before incorporating it into a unit. I was able to take it and work with people in my caseload. Once I become aware and proficient about when and where to introduce it, I could work with my team and introduce them to it. I could educate them into identifying underlying trauma and the best way to assess for it. I could explain how to approach it, how to understand the associational chain and teach it to patients and so on. Because I really understood it well, it enabled me to communicate with my team and promoted our ability to operate as a team to support the patients. I am a certified TIR level one trainer and am also willing to consult to and support individuals and organizations seeking to establish a similar program into an existing health care practice.

Victor: How does TIR change when you are working with children?

Patricia: I look at the level of their attention span. I find that the sessions tend to be shorter with children, generally speaking. I find that there isn't a significant difference in how I do TIR. I take a lot of time in teaching them what to expect. As with adults, I talk about the process of TIR work and the feelings, thoughts, and sensations that arise. I find that that helps children and adults a lot by knowing what to expect. I find it a similar process for each. I'm just more cautious about the age of the child and their ability to sustain focused attention.

Victor: Do you find the end points to be similar or different between children and adults?

Patricia: You know, it really can be similar or different. I find that there are very wise children who will reveal incredible insights. Some parents never have an insight they can identify, and vice-versa. It really depends on the individual. I don't find that age is the determinant; rather, each person comes with his or her own level of ability to verbalize, to release things and to be insightful. Sometimes I see differences between males and females in terms of expression. I find that people are unique in that they each bring their own abilities to bear on the issue being addressed. One of the most exciting things about TIR is that it's like a journey that unfolds and you just don't know how it'll look at the end. The other very exciting thing is that in hearing the person's process, you can actually see where an anxiety disorder began or where the tendency toward depression existed. It's almost as if it gets decoded as the individual goes through the session and it's most instructive as to how mental health does and doesn't work for people.

It's also a phenomenal educational experience for the therapist. I believe that all students who are interested should actually learn TIR so they can learn about mental health through that process because it is absolutely more instructive than anything you get at school.

Victor: Thank you for your time and insights.

Part III:

Background and Theory

14	Critical Issues in Trauma Resolution
	by Frank A. Gerbode, M.D.

Adapted from lecture notes of the above mentioned seminar

About Frank A. Gerbode, M.D.

Dr. Gerbode is an Honors graduate of Stanford University who later pursued graduate studies in philosophy at Cambridge University in England. He received his medical degree from Yale University, and completed a psychiatric residency at Stanford University Medical Center in the early 1970s. Gerbode is the author of numerous papers and articles, which have been published in the *Journal of Neurochemistry*, the *International Journal of Neuropharmacology*, the *Journal of Rational Emotive and Cognitive Behavioral Therapy* and elsewhere. He teaches and lectures internationally, and is the author of *Beyond Psychology: an Introduction to Metapsychology*, now in its 3rd edition.

Traumatic Incident Reduction: A Simple Trauma Resolution Technique

Most common approaches to post-traumatic stress reduction fall into two categories: coping techniques and cathartic techniques. Some therapists give their clients specific in vivo (literally "in life") methods for counteracting or coping with the symptoms of Post-Traumatic Stress Disorder (PTSD), tools to permit their clients to learn to adapt to, to learn to live with, their PTSD condition. Others encourage their clients to release their feelings, to have a catharsis. The idea is that past traumas generate a certain amount of negative energy or "emotional charge", and the therapist's task is to work with the client to release this charge so that it does not manifest itself as aberrant behavior, negative feelings and attitudes, or psychosomatic conditions.

Coping methods and cathartic techniques may help a person to feel better temporarily, but they don't *resolve* trauma so that it can no longer exert a negative effect on the client. Clients feel better temporarily after coping or having a catharsis, but the basic charge remains in place, and shortly thereafter, they need more therapy.

The Need for Anamnesis (recovery of repressed memories)

Traumatic Incident Reduction (TIR) operates on the principle that a permanent resolution of a case requires anamnesis (recovery of re-

pressed memories), rather than mere catharsis or coping. To understand why clients have to achieve an anamnesis in order to resolve past
trauma, we must take a person-centered viewpoint, i.e., the client's
viewpoint. This allows us to explain what makes trauma traumatic.

Time and Intention

Let us start by taking a person-centered look at the subject of time
(see Fig. 14-1). Objectively, we view time as a "never-ending stream", an
undifferentiated continuum in which events are embedded. But subjectively, we actually *experience* time differently. Subjectively, time is
broken up into "chunks" which we shall call "periods" of time. "A time",
for me, is a period during which something was happening or, more
specifically, during which I was doing something, engaging in some activity. Some periods of time are in the past; some are in the present.
Those periods defined by completed activities are in the past; those defined by ongoing (and therefore incomplete) activities are in the present.

The Contents of the Present

For that reason, we don't experience present time as a dimension-
less point. It has breadth corresponding to the width of the activities in
which we are currently engaged. For example, I am still in the period of
time when I was a father, when I was attending this conference, when I
was delivering this workshop, when I was uttering this sentence, when I
was saying this word. These are all activities in which I am engaged,
and each defines a period of time with a definite width. In fact, I inhabit
a host of time periods simultaneously.

Activity Cycles

A period of time has a simple but definite anatomy, determined by
the activity in which you are engaged, which we call an "activity cycle"
or just a "cycle" (See Fig. 14-2). The period of time (and the cycle) starts
when the activity starts, continues as long as the activity continues,
and ends when the activity ends. The activity in question may be related or unrelated to trauma. It could be trying to get away from a
sniper, or it could be vacationing. For instance, the period of time
"when I was going from Paris to Rome" starts when I begin the process
of getting from Paris to Rome, continues while I get the train tickets, get
on the train, and eat in the dining car, and ends when I arrive in Paris.
If an activity has started but not ended for me, that period of time is
still ongoing and is part of my present time.

The Ruling Intention

Moreover, each of my activities is ruled by a governing intention. In the example I just gave, the intention was to get from Paris to Rome but, in the case of a combat veteran, it could be an intention "to get revenge." In effect, therefore, an activity cycle starts when I formulate an intention, continues so long as that intention continues to exist, and only ends when the intention is ended. Therefore, there is an intimate relation between time and intention.

Each of the activities in Fig. 14-1 is coextensive with a corresponding intention. Each continues until the intention is fulfilled or unmade. Present time consists of periods of time that are determined by my current intentions.

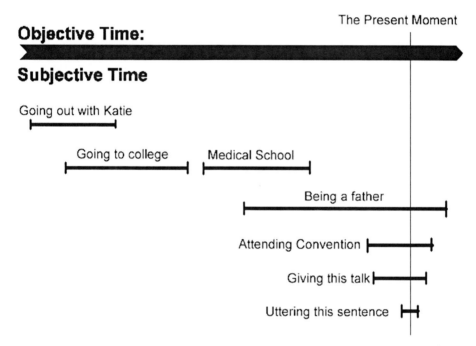

Fig. 14-1: Objective vs. subjective time

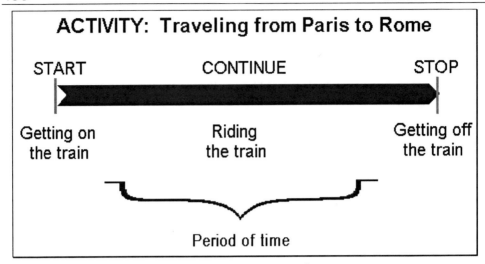

Fig. 14-2: Intention and time

Ending an Intention

In fact, there are only two ways to end an intention and thus to send a period of time into the past:

Fulfill it: An intention ends more or less automatically when it is fulfilled; because you don't keep intending to do things that you know you have already finished doing.

Discontinue it: Even if an intention is not fulfilled, you can deliberately and consciously decide to *unmake* the intention. Unmaking it, however, requires that you be *aware* of it and of your reasons for making it. You cannot unmake an intention of which you are unaware.

In other words, you can't stop doing something you don't know you are doing.

The Effects of Repression

Repressing an incomplete cycle makes it destructive and, at the same time, much more difficult to complete. As mentioned above, to complete a cycle, I must be aware of the intention that rules it. But if, because of the trauma it contains, I have repressed the incident in which I created the intention, I am not aware that I *have* that intention or why I have it, so I cannot unmake it! That period of time continues up into the present, and some energy remains tied up in it. In fact, it makes sense to define charge as "repressed, unfulfilled intention". Getting rid of charge, then, consists of un-repressing intentions and then unmaking them.

Now it becomes obvious why we need anamnesis in order to resolve the effects of past traumas. To reduce the charge contained in past traumas, the client must come fully into contact with them, so that he can find the unfulfilled intentions that he has repressed and why he formulated them, and unmake them.

To Repress or Not to Repress?

Whenever something painful and difficult shows up in life, one has a choice:

1. To allow oneself to experience it fully.

    a. This makes one fully aware of one's intentions in the incident, and why one formed those intentions.
    b. This allows a choice whether or not to unmake the intentions.
    c. At that point, the incident is discharged, by the above definition of "charge", and becomes a *past* incident.

       or

2. To repress it, wholly or partially.

    a. This makes one unaware of the intentions one made in the incident, or why one made them.
    b. This makes it impossible to unmake those intentions.
    c. Thus the incident remains charged and continues on as part of present time.

Paradoxically, by trying to get rid of the incident through repression, one causes it to remain present indefinitely.

Effects of Charge

Charge represents a drain on a person's energy or vitality, because energy remains tied up in the incomplete cycle connected with the intention in the trauma, and more is tied up in the effort to repress the incident. Hence, a person with unresolved past traumas tends to be rather listless or goalless in life. A second effect of past traumas compounds the difficulty: similar conditions in the environment can trigger or "restimulate" past, repressed traumas, just as the sound of a bell could cause Pavlov's dog to salivate. When one is reminded of a past trauma, one has, again, the choice given above: one can either allow oneself to become fully aware of what happened in the original incident or one can repress the incident of being *reminded*. Repression causes the "reminder" incident to become a secondary trauma in itself. Later, similar occurrences can then restimulate the secondary traumatic incident as well as the original one.

A Sequence of Traumatic Incidents

For example (See Fig. 14-3), consider an 8-year-old child who has a past traumatic incident of witnessing her father beating her mother unconscious. Contained in this incident are, say, the feel of the rug, sound of an ambulance, the taste of chewing gum, and, perhaps, other children crying. Also, her parents are arguing loudly and cursing. Since this incident is extremely frightening and traumatic, the child represses it, at least partially. She "doesn't want to think about it."

Later, some years after her parents divorce, her mother and new stepfather have a barbeque in the backyard. She is chewing gum and another child is crying. The two parents are having a loud argument over who knows what. She starts to be reminded consciously or unconsciously of the original incident and feels the fear contained in it. This becomes uncomfortable, so she represses the incident in the backyard, wholly or partly. Contained in it were also the smell of a barbeque and the sound of a dog barking.

In a later incident, she is playing on the living room rug, the scent of the neighbor's barbeque is wafting in the window, the dog barks, and the child suddenly experiences a feeling of fear, because the earlier incident, the one in the backyard, is restimulated by the common elements: the dog barking, the barbeque smell, and the texture of the rug. This is uncomfortable, so she represses this one also, and it becomes another secondary trauma. This incident also contains some additional elements: the sound of the TV and her little brother, playing and talking.

Later, she is trying to fall asleep in her room upstairs. Her little brother is fussing and refuses to calm down. There is shouting downstairs she can hear through the floor but can't quite make out the words. She hears an ambulance approaching the neighborhood. Again, she experiences paralyzing fear because of the reminders, although because the past trauma is repressed, she will attribute the fear to something else, e.g. to the noise of muted shouting or her brother annoying her. This incident contains lying in bed and being afraid to move. It, too, is repressed.

External Restimulators	Icons of Stimuli	Theme (Response)
1. Rug Texture 2. Ambulance 3. Taste of Gum 4. Crying 5. Loud Voices	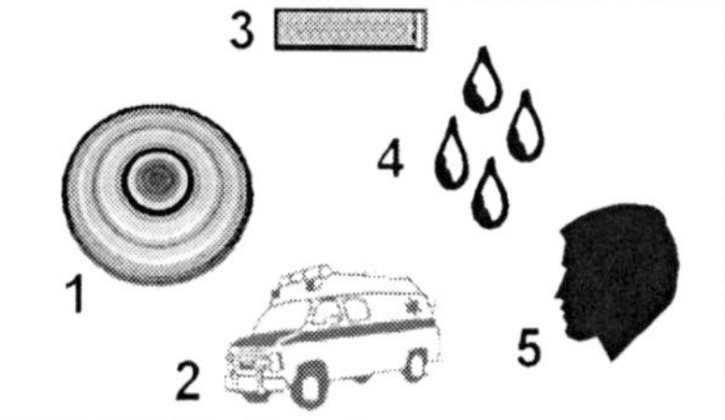	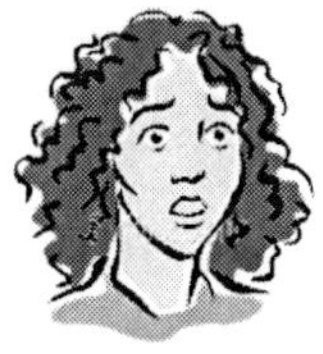 Fear
1. BBQ Smell 2. Dog Barking 3. Taste of Gum 4. Crying 5. Loud Voices	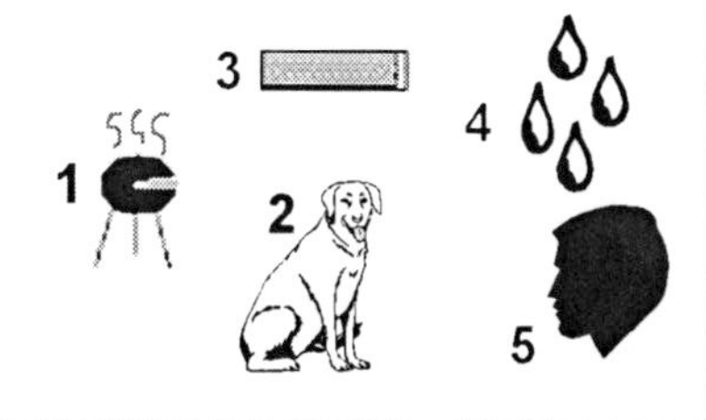	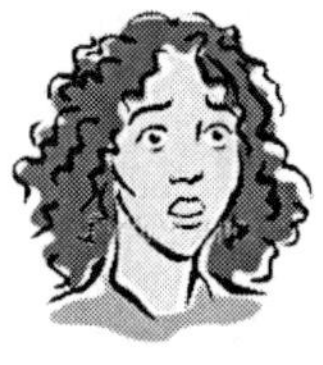 Fear
1. BBQ Smell 2. Dog Barking 3. Rug Texture 4. TV (sound) 5. Little Brother	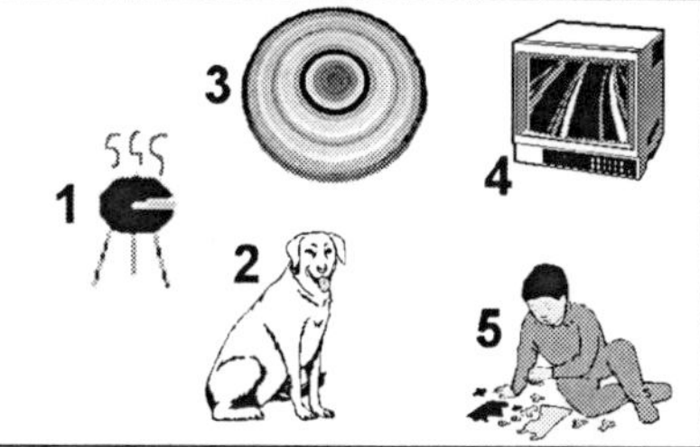	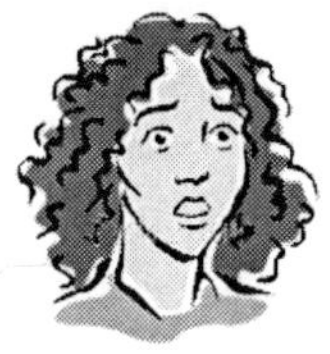 Fear
1. Insomnia 2. Lying in Bed 3. Sirens 4. Loud Voices 5. Little Brother	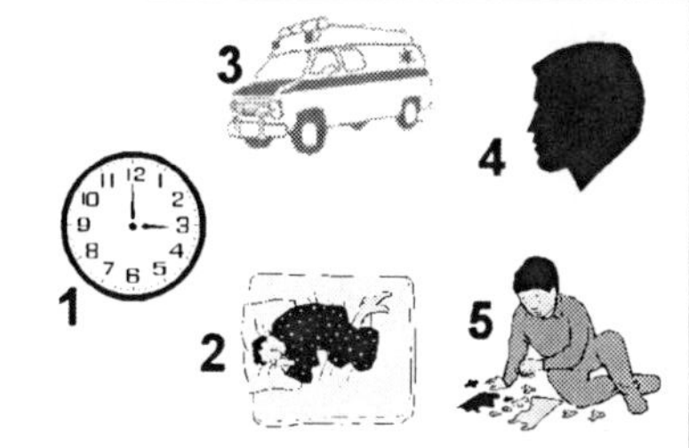	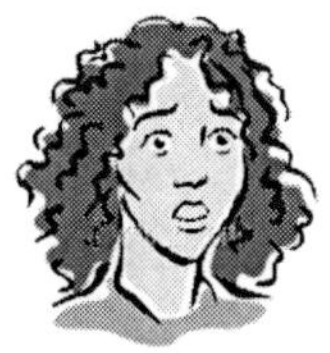 Fear
1. Rug Texture 2. Sirens 3. Lemonade 4. TV (sound) 5. Little Brother	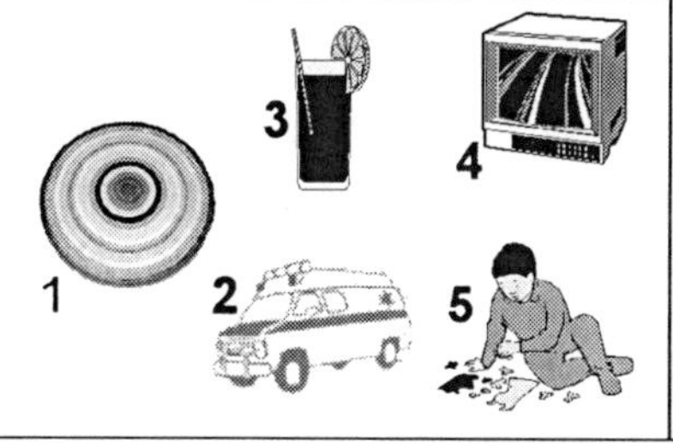	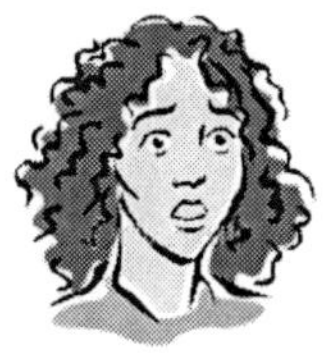 Fear

Fig. 14–3: A sequence of traumatic incidents

Later still, she is drinking lemonade, sitting on the rug, watching TV with her brother, and sirens are in the far distance. The sounds of TV and sirens, and being with her brother trigger the earlier incident and she feels fear. Now, whenever she is on the rug or watching television, she feels unaccountable fear. Her mother gets upset that she won't drink lemonade anymore. Random dream elements further restimulate the same sequence of traumas, resulting in recurring nightmares. Finally, she cannot function at school and is found to be a full-blown PTSD case.

This is a sequence of traumatic incidents, starting with a "root" incident and encompassing, probably, a large number of subsequent incidents in which the root incident or one of its related incidents got restimulated. The only thing in common to all these incidents is the feeling of being scared that she experiences each time. She attributes this fear to something in present time, but it actually stems from the original fright she felt in the root incident.

The Traumatic Incident Network

Although we have only shown a few incidents, in real life a sequence may contain hundreds or even thousands of incidents. Furthermore, the average person usually has a fairly large number of these sequences, with different themes in common. These sequences overlap each other to form a network of traumatic incidents, which we call the traumatic incident network or "Net" (See Fig. 14-4). The object of TIR is to reduce the amount of charge the Net contains so that the person is not subject to the restimulating effects described above, and also so that he can reclaim the intention units that are tied up in the Net.

What we have shown here is not just the situation of a child witness of domestic violence or a rape survivor. It is the human condition. Every one of us has had some past traumas that cause us to be dysfunctional in certain areas of life, the ones that contain restimulators.

The Solution to the Net

Stating the solution is easy, but accomplishing it is somewhat trickier. Traumas contain very intense, repressed, unfulfilled intentions, such as the intention to get revenge, to escape and, of course, the intention to repress the incident. The client needs to find the root incident for each sequence and bring it to full awareness. Traumatic Incident Reduction accomplishes this result. When that occurs, the person becomes aware of the intentions in them and, since these intentions are generally no longer relevant to the here and now, she unmakes them. At that point, the cycles contained in the incidents are completed; they become part of the past, and they can no longer be restimulated.

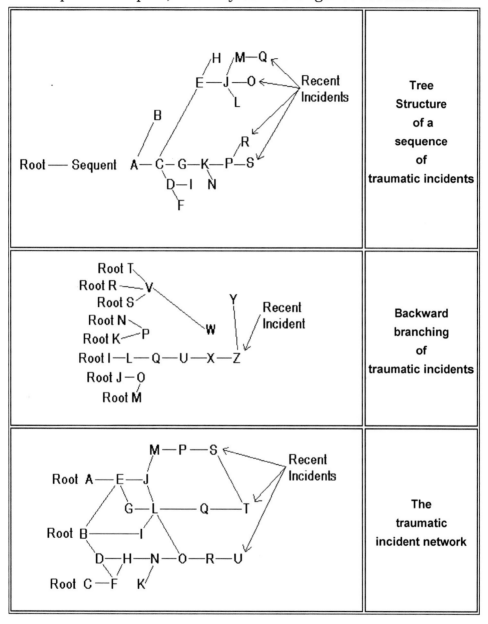

Fig. 14–4: The Traumatic Incident Network

Undoing Amnesia

What is required, then, to obtain the necessary anamnesis? An incident has four dimensions, not just three. In order to be aware of an incident, it is necessary to start at the beginning and go through to the end, like viewing a motion picture, not like looking at a snapshot. Hence, we call the procedure "viewing", the client a "viewer", and we call the one who helps the client to do the viewing the "facilitator". [For more explanation of these terms, please see the glossary beginning on p. 135]

You can't just glance at a part of an incident and expect thereby to have fully completed the process of anamnesis, because you will miss other parts of it—probably the most important ones, the ones that are most difficult to confront. In order to achieve a full anamnesis, you must be allowed to go through the entire incident without interruptions, without reassurances, in short without *any* distractions. Furthermore, it does not suffice to go through the incident only once. If you want to become fully familiar with a movie, you must see it a number of times, and each time you will notice new things about it. The same thing happens during Traumatic Incident Reduction, except that the client is viewing a past traumatic incident instead of a movie, and that's somewhat harder to do.

Basic vs. Thematic TIR

If, as is often the case with combat vets and rape victims—survivors of single or discrete incidents—the viewer already knows which trauma needs to be looked at, you can use a relatively simple form of TIR called "Basic TIR". You simply have the viewer go through the single, known incident enough times to resolve it. But in most cases, the viewer starts out being entirely unaware of what the root trauma underlying his difficulties is. So how can he find it? For that, we use a technique called "Thematic TIR", in which we can trace back an unwanted feeling, emotion, sensation, attitude, or pain to the original root trauma.

End Points

When the viewer finds and discharges the root incident, a very specific and often quite dramatic series of phenomena appear, showing that the viewer has achieved a thorough discharge. Then we say that the viewer has reached an "end point." These phenomena usually appear in the following order in adults:

1. *Positive indicators*: The viewer appears happy, relieved, or serene. She is not sitting in the middle of something heavy. Sometimes she will laugh or say something cheerful. In the absence of good indicators, a full end point has not occurred.

2. *Realization*: Then the viewer will usually voice some kind of realization or insight, a reflection of the fact that he is becoming more aware.

3. *Extroversion*: Finally, the viewer will open her eyes or otherwise indicate that her attention is now back in the present. She will usually look at the facilitator or at the room, or make some comment about something in the here and now.

4. *Intention and/or decision made at the time of the incident expressed*: Often, the viewer will explicitly tell the facilitator what intention was present in the incident. If he doesn't, the facilitator has the option of asking him to tell of any decisions he may have made at the time of the incident.

In children, instead of such positive indicators, you may find that they simply tend to lose interest in the incident. They will stop being fixated on it. Also, children are less likely to report realizations, perhaps since they have a shorter train of baggage tied to the incident.

When you see an end point, the most important thing to do is to stop. If you continue past the point when the root incident has been discharged, and continue to ask the viewer to look for incidents, she will start to wander around more or less randomly in the Net, and will often end up triggering a lot of things that you may not be able to resolve with TIR, at least in the framework of one session. This is called an *overrun*.

Flows

A person can have charge, not only on what has been done to him but also on what he has done to others, what others have done to others, and what he has done to himself. These are actually four principal directions in which causation can flow:

Inflow:	From something or someone in the world outside.
Outflow:	From the viewer to others. These are things the viewer has done, inadvertently or on purpose, that have affected others. Handling this flow tends to alleviate guilt.
Crossflow:	To others, but not from the viewer, i.e., from something in the world outside or from other people to others. The viewer is "only a spectator" here; nevertheless, such incidents can be very heavily charged, as in the case of a mother witnessing her child being threatened or hurt.
Reflexive flow:	From self to self.

When a viewer has a charged incident that contains one of these flows, it is quite possible, even likely, that she will also have similar incidents on other flows that are also charged. After a viewer addresses an incident in which she was betrayed, the facilitator may ask if there were any incidents in which she betrayed another, and also whether there is charge on one or more incidents in which she observed others being betrayed. There may even be incidents in which, as she perceives it, she betrayed herself.

As a person comes up in awareness, he tends first to be aware of what others have done to him, then of what he has done to others, then of what others have done to others, and finally, what he has done to himself. Both Basic and Thematic TIR instructions can and should consider flows.

Results

We have found that TIR works well with most clients who fit the criteria for PTSD. An exception is that TIR does not work well with people who are currently abusing drugs or alcohol. When the viewer has been drinking heavily or abusing other substances between sessions, it will fail virtually every time. Another contraindication is if the client is diagnosable with some type of personality disorder.

Although the TIR procedure is not complicated or difficult to learn, it can only work in a session environment that is structured in such a way that it is safe. Much of the TIR training involves teaching certain Rules of Facilitation and communication skills specific to the TIR style of working with a client.

<table>
<tr><td>15</td><td>

PTSD in Children and Adolescents

by Jessica Hamblen PhD

A National Center for PTSD Fact Sheet

</td></tr>
</table>

The diagnosis of Posttraumatic Stress Disorder (PTSD) was formally recognized as a psychiatric diagnosis in 1980. At that time, little was known about what PTSD looked like in children and adolescents. Today, we know children and adolescents are susceptible to developing PTSD, and we know that PTSD has different age-specific features. In addition, we are beginning to develop child-focused interventions. This fact sheet provides information regarding what events cause PTSD in children, how many children develop PTSD, risk factors associated with PTSD, what PTSD looks like in children, other effects of trauma on children, treatment for PTSD, and what you can do for your child.

What events cause PTSD in children?

A diagnosis of PTSD means that an individual experienced an event that involved a threat to one's own or another's life or physical integrity and that this person responded with intense fear, helplessness, or horror. There are a number of traumatic events that have been shown to cause PTSD in children and adolescents. Children and adolescents may be diagnosed with PTSD if they have survived natural and man made disasters such as floods; violent crimes such as kidnapping, rape or murder of a parent, sniper fire, and school shootings; motor vehicle accidents such as automobile and plane crashes; severe burns; exposure to community violence; war; peer suicide; and sexual and physical abuse.

How many children develop PTSD?

A few studies of the general population have been conducted that examine rates of exposure and PTSD in children and adolescents . Results from these studies indicate that 15 to 43% of girls and 14 to 43% of boys have experienced at least one traumatic event in their lifetime. Of those children and adolescents who have experienced a trauma, 3 to 15% of girls and 1 to 6% of boys could be diagnosed with PTSD.

Rates of PTSD are much higher in children and adolescents recruited from at-risk samples. The rates of PTSD in these at-risk children and adolescents vary from 3 to 100%. For example, studies have shown that as many as 100% of children who witness a parental homicide or sexual assault develop PTSD. Similarly, 90% of sexually abused children, 77% of children exposed to a school shooting, and 35% of urban youth exposed to community violence develop PTSD.

What are the risk factors for PTSD?

There are three factors that have been shown to increase the likelihood that children will develop PTSD. These factors include the severity of the traumatic event, the parental reaction to the traumatic event, and the physical proximity to the traumatic event. In general, most studies find that children and adolescents who report experiencing the most severe traumas also report the highest levels of PTSD symptoms. Family support and parental coping have also been shown to affect PTSD symptoms in children. Studies show that children and adolescents with greater family support and less parental distress have lower levels of PTSD symptoms. Finally, children and adolescents who are farther away from the traumatic event report less distress.

There are several other factors that affect the occurrence and severity of PTSD. Research suggests that interpersonal traumas such as rape and assault are more likely to result in PTSD than other types of traumas. Additionally, if an individual has experienced a number of traumatic events in the past, those experiences increase the risk of developing PTSD. In terms of gender, several studies suggest that girls are more likely than boys to develop PTSD. A few studies have examined the connection between ethnicity and PTSD. While some studies find that minorities report higher levels of PTSD symptoms, researchers have shown that this is due to other factors such as differences in levels of exposure. It is not clear how a child's age at the time of exposure to a traumatic event impacts the occurrence or severity of PTSD. While some studies find a relationship, others do not. Differences that do occur may be due to differences in the way PTSD is expressed in children and adolescents of different ages or developmental levels (see next section).

What does PTSD look like in children?

Researchers and clinicians are beginning to recognize that PTSD may not present itself in children the same way it does in adults (see *What is PTSD?* below). Criteria for PTSD now include age-specific features for some symptoms.

Very young children may present with few PTSD symptoms. This may be because eight of the PTSD symptoms require a verbal descrip-

tion of one's feelings and experiences. Instead, young children may report more generalized fears such as stranger or separation anxiety,
avoidance of situations that may or may not be related to the trauma,
sleep disturbances, and a preoccupation with words or symbols that
may or may not be related to the trauma. These children may also dis-
play posttraumatic play in which they repeat themes of the trauma. In
addition, children may lose an acquired developmental skill (such as
toilet training) as a result of experiencing a traumatic event.

Clinical reports suggest that elementary school-aged children may
not experience visual flashbacks or amnesia for aspects of the trauma.
However, they do experience "time skew" and "omen formation," which
are not typically seen in adults. Time skew refers to a child mis-
sequencing trauma related events when recalling the memory. Omen
formation is a belief that there were warning signs that predicted the
trauma. As a result, children often believe that if they are alert enough,
they will recognize warning signs and avoid future traumas. School-
aged children also reportedly exhibit posttraumatic play or reenactment
of the trauma in play, drawings, or verbalizations. Posttraumatic play is
different from reenactment in that posttraumatic play is a literal representation of the trauma, involves compulsively repeating some aspect of
the trauma, and does not tend to relieve anxiety. An example of post-
traumatic play is an increase in shooting games after exposure to a
school shooting. Posttraumatic reenactment, on the other hand, is more
flexible and involves behaviorally recreating aspects of the trauma (e.g.,
carrying a weapon after exposure to violence).

PTSD in adolescents may begin to more closely resemble PTSD in
adults. However, there are a few features that have been shown to dif-
fer. As discussed above, children may engage in traumatic play
following a trauma. Adolescents are more likely to engage in traumatic
reenactment, in which they incorporate aspects of the trauma into their
daily lives. In addition, adolescents are more likely than younger children or adults to exhibit impulsive and aggressive behaviors.

Besides PTSD, what are the other effects of trauma on children?

Besides PTSD, children and adolescents who have experienced
traumatic events often exhibit other types of problems. Perhaps the
best information available on the effects of traumas on children comes
from a review of the literature on the effects of child sexual abuse. In
this review, it was shown that sexually abused children often have
problems with fear, anxiety, depression, anger and hostility, aggression,

sexually inappropriate behavior, self-destructive behavior, feelings of isolation and stigma, poor self-esteem, difficulty in trusting others, and substance abuse. These problems are often seen in children and adolescents who have experienced other types of traumas as well. Children who have experienced traumas also often have relationship problems with peers and family members, problems with acting out, and problems with school performance.

Along with associated symptoms, there are a number of psychiatric disorders that are commonly found in children and adolescents who have been traumatized. One commonly co-occurring disorder is major depression. Other disorders include substance abuse; other anxiety disorders such as separation anxiety, panic disorder, and generalized anxiety disorder; and externalizing disorders such as Attention-Deficit/Hyperactivity Disorder, oppositional defiant disorder, and conduct disorder.

How is PTSD treated in children and adolescents?

Although some children show a natural remission in PTSD symptoms over a period of a few months, a significant number of children continue to exhibit symptoms for years if untreated. Few treatment studies have examined which treatments are most effective for children and adolescents. A review of the adult treatment studies of PTSD shows that Cognitive-Behavioral Therapy (CBT) is the most effective approach. CBT for children generally includes the child directly discussing the traumatic event (exposure), anxiety management techniques such as relaxation and assertiveness training, and correction of inaccurate or distorted trauma related thoughts. Although there is some controversy regarding exposing children to the events that scare them, exposure-based treatments seem to be most relevant when memories or reminders of the trauma distress the child. Children can be exposed gradually and taught relaxation so that they can learn to relax while recalling their experiences. Through this procedure, they learn that they do not have to be afraid of their memories. CBT also involves challenging children's false beliefs such as, "the world is totally unsafe." The majority of studies have found that it is safe and effective to use CBT for children with PTSD.

CBT is often accompanied by psychoeducation and parental involvement. Psychoeducation is education about PTSD symptoms and their effects. It is as important for parents and caregivers to understand the effects of PTSD as it is for children. Research shows that the better parents cope with the trauma, and the more they support their children, the better their children will function. Therefore, it is important for parents to seek treatment for themselves in order to develop the necessary coping skills that will help their children.

Several other types of therapy have been suggested for PTSD in children and adolescents. Play therapy can be used to treat young children with PTSD who are not able to deal with the trauma more directly. The therapist uses games, drawings, and other techniques to help the children process their traumatic memories. Psychological first aid has been prescribed for children exposed to community violence and can be used in schools and traditional settings. Psychological first aid involves clarifying trauma related facts, normalizing the children's PTSD reactions, encouraging the expression of feelings, teaching problem solving skills, and referring the most symptomatic children for additional treatment. Twelve Step approaches have been prescribed for adolescents with substance abuse problems and PTSD. Another therapy, Eye Movement Desensitization and Reprocessing (EMDR), combines cognitive therapy with directed eye movements. While EMDR has been shown to be effective in treating both children and adults with PTSD, studies indicate that it is the cognitive intervention rather than the eye movements that accounts for the change. Medications have also been prescribed for some children with PTSD. However, due to the lack of research in this area, it is too early to evaluate the effectiveness of medication therapy.

Finally, specialized interventions may be necessary for children exhibiting particularly problematic behaviors or PTSD symptoms. For example, a specialized intervention might be required for inappropriate sexual behavior or extreme behavioral problems.

What can I do to help my child?

Reading this fact sheet is a first step toward helping your child. Gather information on PTSD and pay attention to how your child is functioning. Watch for warning signs such as sleep problems, irritability, avoidance, changes in school performance, and problems with peers. It may be necessary to seek help for your child. Consider having your child evaluated by a mental-health professional who has experience treating PTSD in children and adolescents. Ask how the therapist typically treats PTSD, and choose a practitioner with whom you and your child feel comfortable. Consider whether you might also benefit from talking to someone individually. The most important thing you can do now is to support your child.

This document is based in part on the "Practice Parameters for the Assessment and Treatment of Children and Adolescents with Posttraumatic Stress Disorder", *Journal of the American Academy of Child and Adolescent Psychiatry*, 37:10 supplement, October 1998.

Glossary

Basic TIR: The application of TIR to specific, known traumatic incidents.

Case Plan: The written plan of viewing techniques, designed using data from an interview to accomplish the viewer's goals for viewing.

Case Planning: The action of deciding which techniques should be used with a client and the order in which they should be done.

Charge: Repressed, unfulfilled intention. Charge attached to an issue is experienced as a feeling of resistance, physical or emotional pain or unpleasantness, or lessened consciousness.

Communication Exercises: Exercises to improve a facilitator's skill in each aspect of communication in a viewing session.

End Point: The point at which a viewing procedure (or other activity) is completed. In viewing, it consists of extroversion of the viewer's attention, positive or very positive indicators, and often a realization of some kind.

Engagement: In viewing, the state in which the viewer is attentive to an item of charged case material and, using a viewing procedure and the help of the facilitator, is actively working through the item to discharge and resolve it.

Exploration: TIR and similar formal techniques have predetermined questions. *Exploration* is asking questions that are not part of these techniques. We name this as a technique in itself in order to maintain the integrity of the person-centered context of the work. Each Exploration has its own end point, depending on what we intend to accomplish with it, for example: sorting out something confusing that arises during a session, or addressing an area of interest in order to remove charge from it.

Facilitation: The act of helping another person (viewer) to perform the actions of viewing.

Facilitator: A practitioner of TIR and Metapsychology.

Fixed Idea: An idea that a viewer adheres to because it keeps the viewer from having to face up to something such as a painful situation, a confusion, or problem.

Flat Point: A point at which a viewing procedure can safely be stopped without leaving the viewer in heavy charge; a minor End Point. In training, a point at which the student (trainee) is no longer reacting to a button.

Flows: A direction of causation between people, or people and entities (things). The flows commonly addressed in viewing are: inflow, outflow, cross-flow (another to another) and reflexive flow (self to self).

Future TIR (FTIR): A special application of TIR to remove charge from future events, whether probable or improbable, that the viewer is concerned about.

Grounding techniques: Techniques used to destimulate and stabilize an overwhelmed viewer, or to ground a viewer in preparation for ending the session if a full End Point cannot be reached in that session. (See Locational Remedies)

Indication: A deliberate assertion about something related to a person's case, personality, situation or condition. A *right* or *correct indication* would be one that resonates as true to the person receiving it. Compare with *Wrong indication.*

Indicator(s): Visible manifestations that indicate how a viewer is doing. Positive indicators include extroversion, viewer looking brighter, smiles, laughter, and realizations. Negative indicators include any viewer manifestations of dissatisfaction with the session or facilitator.

Life Stress Reduction: A case plan written for an individual viewer for the purpose of addressing and discharging case material currently in restimulation of interest to that viewer. The end point of Life Stress Reduction is a viewer feeling destimulated, cheerful, extroverted and ready to tackle life anew.

Locational Remedies: Relatively brief techniques meant to assist a person to a more comfortable state by directing the viewer's attention to objects in the environment, without necessarily causing significant change in the person's condition.

Loop(s): A set of questions to be used over and over in sequence until an end point is reached. Depending on the number of questions, it would be called a "2-part loop," a "3-part loop," and so forth.

Metapsychology (Often used to mean Applied Metapsychology, as used in facilitation/viewing sessions): The person-centered application of techniques designed to permit the viewer to examine his or her: life, mind, emotions, experiences (including traumatic experiences), decisions, fixed ideas and successes. It has the aim of resolving areas of charge and returning the viewer to a better condition, in the person's own estimation.

Remedies: Relatively brief techniques meant to assist a viewer to a more comfortable state without necessarily causing significant change in the person's condition.

Restimulation: An instance of charged material, such as a sequence of traumatic incidents, being activated so that the person feels effects from it, knowingly or unknowingly.

Technical Direction: The action of writing individualized case plans for facilitators to use with viewers as well as written directions of how to proceed from one session to the next; also used to mean such a written direction for a session (also called a session agenda).

Technique: (also sometimes "procedure"): A pattern of viewing instructions designed to address a certain type of charged case material (such as Traumatic Incidents, upsets, charge on a specific person, etc.) and meant to be continued to an End Point.

Thematic TIR: A form of TIR that deals with sequences of traumatic incidents, all of which have a certain theme in common, and traces them back to the first trauma in the sequence, or root incident.

Theme: A common element that the different traumatic incidents in a sequence all have in common. Themes are negative feelings, emotions, sensations, attitudes and pains.

Touch Remedy: A Remedy that directs the viewer's attention to various points through the body in order to restore communication with the body. This can be used to calm a distraught viewer, for grounding, or for reducing physical discomfort.

Unblocking: A procedure in which a number of mental blocks on a certain issue are addressed repetitively until charge has been reduced on that subject. See the following page for a fuller description.

Unlayering: A type of procedure involving one or many repetitive viewing instructions.

Viewer: The client in viewing session.

Wrong Indication: An evaluative and generally invalidative statement that violates the recipient's self-concept and perception of truth; also see "Indication".

A Brief Description of Unblocking

Unblocking uses the method called *unlayering,* which involves the use of a question or set of questions asked repetitively until an end point is reached. Unlayering allows a client to look at a particular area of life many separate times, thus peeling off layers of thoughts, considerations, emotions, decisions, and opinions. Each time the question is asked, the viewer gets a new look at the subject until there are no more answers to that question.

Unblocking, a special application of unlayering, consists of numerous questions that have been tested and proven to be the most useful in helping a client uncover and remove charge from a significant issue. This is a thorough enough technique that we don't want to use it on a very minor issue, but rather something central to the person's life.

Some real life examples of areas addressed effectively with Unblocking:

- your self-esteem (or: how you feel about yourself)
- how other people feel about you
- your self confidence
- your possessions
- school
- your relationship with (charged persons such as "your mother" or "your friends")
- your neighborhood
- your hobbies

Unblocking has the advantage of being less challenging for the client and so is often used to prepare a client for being able to use TIR, but it should not be relegated to a category of TIR preparation alone. It has great value in allowing us to address issues that may not have traumatic incidents connected to them, but are still worrisome and absorbing to the client.

TIR is what we call a "checklist technique" because it consists of a series of steps the client is asked to do in order, each of which build upon the ones that went before. Repetition comes into it in that the client is allowed to go through the incident in question as many times as needed to either bring about resolution or to allow an earlier related incident to come into view. Because the viewer is being asked to go back and re-experience a traumatic incident in TIR, it is fairly demanding on the client (though well worth the effort).

Unblocking allows the client to look at whatever comes up in response to the question, in whatever order it comes up. End points reported by clients on Unblocking include such things as greater clarity and understanding of that area of life, and a greater certainty.

Memory Lists for Children
by Hildegard Jahn

Introduction

Memory Lists serve several functions in Applied Metapsychology. For example, they can be used to build confidence and skill in the basic viewing procedures when used with a new client. For fragile clients who are not yet ready for Traumatic Incident Reduction or even Unblocking, memory lists provide an access to pleasure incidents.

Anecdotally, there are two common outcomes associated with successful use of memory lists. First, the past becomes more accessible—in the sense that it is less of a thing to be feared. Second, the ability to recall details and even whole time periods generally improves. In that sense, memory is a kind of muscle that improves with use.

Although the Memory Lists can be used in any order, the Remedial Recall List is specially designed to be helpful following techniques which have failed to reach a good end point.

Instructions

Ask each question once, and then ask for an earlier instance, then the earliest the child can remember of each question. If this is too much for the child you are working with, just ask each question once, allowing the child to tell you as much as s/he wants to about each.

1. Plants and Animals

Can you remember a time when:
1. You have seen an animal?
2. A cat was purring?
3. You planted something?
4. You gathered fruits or berries and ate them?
5. You found out that an animal liked you?
6. It was wonderful lying or playing in the grass?
7. You smelled a flower?
8. You listened to a bird?
9. You felt that a tree was beautiful?
10. You felt that it was wonderful to walk through a large meadow?
11. An animal came close to you?
12. You knew just what an animal thought or felt?
13. An animal understood what you wanted?
14. You eagerly observed an insect?
15. You gently touched an animal?
16. It was beautiful to be in the shadow of a tree?
17. You heard a bird sing?
18. You strolled with friends through a forest?
19. You found out that an animal was intelligent?
20. You went into a zoo?
21. You fed an animal?
22. You observed a fish?
23. You spoke with an animal?
24. An animal acted in a very funny way?
25. You cared for a plant?
26. You picked flowers?

Knowledge, Training, Learning

Can you remember a time when:
1. You learned something that impressed you?
2. Somebody taught you in something in a very nice way?
3. You found out something by yourself?
4. You painted or drew something?
5. Somebody told you that you are intelligent?
6. You found out by yourself that you are capable of understanding something?
7. You grasped how a toy works?
8. You read a book, or looked at the pictures in a book?
9. Somebody helped you in writing?
10. You were the only one who knew something?
11. You helped someone else learn something?
12. You made a poem?
13. You sang a song?
14. You won a game?
15. Something was difficult to do and you were able to do it?
16. Someone approved of something you built or created?
17. Others noticed that you were right?
18. You were very glad to do something new?
19. You made or did something others did not know that you could do?
20. You had a great pleasure playing with friends?
21. You observed something that moved very quickly?
22. Others told you that you were smart?
23. You found out that your body had grown?
24. You read the time on a clock?
25. You found out that another season had come up?
26. You found out that someone was smaller than you?

Feelings, Emotions, Other Persons

Can you remember a time when:

1. Somebody told you that he/she loves or likes you?
2. Somebody admired you?
3. Someone enjoyed listening to what you said?
4. You shared a secret with someone?
5. You helped or supported someone?
6. Somebody became your friend?
7. You were with friends in a pool, lake, or ocean?
8. You were sledding with friends?
9. You had a ball-game with friends?
10. You and your friend(s) set up a prank to surprise others?
11. You told the truth and felt wonderful?
12. You told someone you love or like him/her?
13. Somebody felt lucky because you helped or supported him/her?
14. A voice was very familiar to you?
15. Somebody felt very cosy with you?
16. Somebody read or told you a story?
17. You were reconciled with someone after having had a quarrel?
18. Someone defended you?
19. You read or told someone a story?
20. You enjoyed it when others were nice to each other?
21. You defended someone against others?
22. You hugged someone?
23. You felt that someone was extremely beautiful?
24. Somebody gave you a present?
25. Someone familiar with you recognised your voice in the dark?
26. Someone was near to you when you needed help and supported you?
27. Someone said that you are good-looking?
28. You recognised the handwriting of someone familiar to you?
29. You liked to kiss or hug someone?
30. You watched TV with someone?
31. You were out of breath in a game?
32. You liked or loved someone you observed in TV?
33. Somebody you liked or admired taught you something?
34. You taught something to someone younger than you?
35. You made someone laugh?
36. Someone praised you?
37. Your group won a game?
38. You had a wonderful birthday party?
39. You disguised yourself in a special costume?

40. You made a journey?
41. You had a picnic with friends/family?
42. You were in a bathtub with others?
43. You did what you promised?
44. Somebody made you laugh?
45. You made a joke?
46. You felt strong?
47. Somebody played a noisy game with you?
48. Somebody helped you to find something?
49. Others were positively astonished about you?
50. A calm voice felt kind to you?
51. You prepared something to eat with someone?
52. You were dressed very handsomely/beautifully?

Things and Surroundings

Can you remember a time when...
1. You rode a bicycle?
2. You were swimming?
3. You made something well as part of a hobby?
4. Running was a pleasure for you?
5. You rearranged things in your own room?
6. You cleverly hid yourself?
7. You knew exactly what you were doing?
8. You felt yourself wonderful in your clothes?
9. Something smelled wonderful?
10. You felt that a machine was fantastic?
11. You had enough space of your own?
12. You had enough time?
13. You had enough to eat?
14. You slid down a hill and it was fun?
15. You played in the water?
16. You found a good place to go skating?
17. You observed something very carefully?
18. Something tasted very good to you?
19. You discovered something that you never saw before?
20. You found something that seemed valuable to you?
21. You listened to marvellous music?
22. You heard a loud and pleasant noise?
23. You were swinging?
24. The wind was blowing intensely?
25. You heard something in the far distance?
26. It was cosy in the dark?
27. You touched something smooth?
28. You ate something you never ate before?
29. You smelled something you never smelled before?
30. You played with something that made music or a pleasant noise?
31. You repaired something?
32. You destroyed something that needed to be destroyed?
33. You found some material you needed in order to make something?

Remedial Recall List for Children

Recommended for use when a session must complete without having reached a good end point.

Can you remember a time when...

1. You made something with another person?
2. You really liked someone?
3. You had a good time communicating with someone?
4. Another person asked you for advice?
5. Someone really liked you?
6. Someone understood you very well?
7. Someone hugged you?
8. Someone cheered you up?
9. You understood someone very well?
10. You cheered someone up?
11. Someone was glad you were there?
12. You knew that you were right?
13. You were happy that someone was coming to see you?
14. Another person was happy that you were coming to see her/him?
15. You liked the feel of something in your hand?
16. You took care of someone so that he/she felt better?
17. You felt cosy and safe?
18. You ate something wonderful?
19. You were surprised and pleased by someone?
20. The moon and the stars were shining beautifully?
21. The sun warmed you?
22. You ran fast just for the fun of it?
23. You were happy to lie down and rest?

Appendix	Information on Receiving
B	**Training in TIR**

Your local trainer may choose to provide co-sponsored trainings that are approved for continuing education. Please look for the following statements in training announcements:

> This program is co-sponsored by Applied Metapsychology International (AMI) and your local trainer. AMI is approved by the American Psychological Association to offer continuing education for psychologists. AMI maintains responsibility for the program and its contents.
>
> This program was approved by the National Association of Social Workers (provider # 886415259) for up to 28 continuing education contact hours.

In addition, all three of the TIR related workshops are approved by the Association of Traumatic Stress Specialists (ATSS) for credit toward their certification programs and for continuing education credit.

The Canadian Counselling Association has recognized each of the three TIR workshops for 4 CEUs. Please notify your trainer in advance if you will require an application for CCA CEUs for a workshop you will be attending.

Three short workshops provide full training in Traumatic Incident Reduction and Life Stress Reduction:

- The TIR Workshop, Level One
- TIR – Expanded Applications
- Case Planning for TIR and Life Stress Reduction

After the first workshop, you will be able to use TIR. For ideal results, you may take the other two workshops in either order. They will expand your use of TIR and provide an array of other techniques to address not only traumatic stress, but also many other issues.

Most trainers also offer follow-up supervision and/or internships for certification.

Beyond Life Stress Reduction (using the techniques taught on the first three workshops), lies the realm of Applied Metapsychology, utilizing similar techniques for personal growth and realizing ones potential.

See the *www.tirtraining.org* website for further information including the Training Calendar. Click on the name of the trainer or contact person for the training you wish to attend and you will be able to send an email for details of that training such as cost and location. Some of the trainers are willing to travel, if you would like to arrange a workshop in your area.

<table>
<tr><td>Appendix

C</td><td># Additional Reading on TIR
and Metapsychology</td></tr>
</table>

Dissertations on or Involving TIR

- Bisbey, L., (1995). "No Longer a Victim: A Treatment Outcome Study of Crime Victims with Post-Traumatic Stress Disorder." (Doctoral Dissertation, California School of Professional Psychology, San Diego, CA.)
  [Ed. Note: Her dissertation compared TIR and Imaginal Flooding with a control group with 57 subjects]
  Specify Order Number 9522269
- Coughlin, W., (1995). "Traumatic Incident Reduction: Efficacy in Reducing Anxiety Symptomatology." (Doctoral Dissertation, Union Institute, Cincinnati, OH.) Specify Order Number 9537919
- Odio, Francine (2003) "Traumatic Incident Reduction (TIR) Program for Children." (Doctoral Dissertation, Carlos Albizu University.) Publication Number AAT 3100829 from Digital Dissertations
- Valentine, Pamela V. (1997) "Traumatic Incident Reduction: Brief Treatment of Trauma-Related Symptoms in Incarcerated Females." (Doctoral Dissertation, Florida State University. Advisor: Smith, Thomas E.)
  Specify Order Number 9725020

Students, faculty, staff and researchers can order their own unbound copies of dissertations and theses with express delivery to their home, school or office. Select from over one million titles available from UMI by visiting http://wwwlib.umi.com/dxweb/

Metapsychology/TIR–Related Literature

In order of publication date:

Gerbode, F.A. (1989). *Beyond Psychology: an Introduction to Meta-psychology*, 3rd Ed. (1995) Menlo Park, CA: IRM Press

Moore, R.H. (1992). "Cognitive-Emotive Treatment of the Post-Traumatic Stress Disorder". In W. Dryden and L. Hill (Eds.) *Innovations in Rational-Emotive Therapy*. Newbury Park, CA: Sage Publications

Moore, R.H. (1993). "Innovative Techniques for Practitioners". *The RET Resource Book for Practitioners*. New York, NY: Institute for Rational-Emotive Therapy.

Gerbode, F.A. & Moore, R.H. (1994). "Beliefs and Intentions in RET." *Journal of Rational-Emotive & Cognitive-Behavior Therapy*, Vol. 12, No. 1., Albert Ellis Institute

French, Gerald D., MA, CTS and Harris, Chrys, Ph.D., CTS (1998), *Traumatic Incident Reduction (TIR)*. CRC Press

Bisbey, L., MA, CTS and Bisbey, S. (1999) *Brief Therapy for Post-Traumatic Stress Disorder: Traumatic Incident Reduction and Related Technique*. John Wiley & Sons.

Descilo, Teresa (1999) "Relieving the Traumatic Aspects of Death with Traumatic Incident Reduction and EMDR". In: pp. 153-182; Figley, Charles R [ed.]; *Traumatology of Grieving: Conceptual, Theoretical, and Treatment Foundations*; Philadelphia: Brunner/Mazel,

Gerbode, F.A. (2005). "Traumatic Incident Reduction" in Garrick and Williams [ed.] *Trauma Treatment Techniques: Innovative trends*. New York, NY: Haworth Press.

Volkman, Marian (2005) *Life Skills: Improve the Quality of Your Life with Metapsychology*. Ann Arbor, MI. Loving Healing Press.

Volkman, Victor (2005) *Beyond Trauma: Conversations on Traumatic Incident Reduction, 2nd Ed*. Ann Arbor, MI. Loving Healing Press.

Volkman, Victor (2005) *Traumatic Incident Reduction: Research and Results*. Ann Arbor, MI. Loving Healing Press.

Volkman, Victor (2006) *Traumatic Incident Reduction and Critical Incident Stress Management*. Ann Arbor, MI. Loving Healing Press.

Volkman, Marian (2007) *Children and Traumatic Incident Reduction: Creative and Cognitive Approaches*. Ann Arbor, MI. Loving Healing Press. Volkman, Victor (2005) *Traumatic Incident Reduction: Research and Results.* Ann Arbor, MI. Loving Healing Press.

Volkman, Victor (2008) *Traumatic Incident Reduction: Research and Results.* Ann Arbor, MI. Loving Healing Press.

Selected Journal Articles about TIR

Dietrich, Anne M; Baranowsky, Anna B; Devich-Navarro, Mona; Gentry, J Eric; Harris, Chrys Jay; Figley, Charles R "A review of alternative approaches to the treatment of post traumatic sequelae." *Traumatology,* 6(4): pp. 251-271, December 2000, ISSN: 1534-7656

Figley, Charles R; Carbonnell, Joyce L; Boscarino, Joseph A; Chang, Jeani. "A Clinical Demonstration Model for Assessing the Effectiveness of Therapeutic Interventions: an Expanded Clinical Trials Methodology." *International Journal of Emergency Mental Health,* 1(3): pp. 155-164, Summer 1999

Gallo, Fred P. "Reflections on active ingredients in efficient treatments of PTSD, part 2." *Traumatology,* 2(2): pp. [Article 2], 1996 ISSN: 1534-7656

Mitchels, B. (2003). "Healing the wounds of war and more: an integrative approach to peace--the work of Adam Curle and others with Mir I. Dobro in Upanja, Croatia". *British Journal of Guidance and Counselling,* 31(4), 403-416.

Valentine, P. and Smith, Thomas E. "Evaluating Traumatic Incident Reduction Therapy with Female Inmates: a Randomized Controlled Clinical Trial." *Research on Social Work Practice,* v. 11, no. 1, pp. 40-52, January 2001, ISSN: 1049-7315

Valentine, P. "Traumatic Incident Reduction I: Traumatized Women Inmates: Particulars of Practice and Research", *Journal of Offender Rehabilitation* Vol. 31(3-4): 1-15, 2000

Valentine, P. and Smith, Thomas E. "A Qualitative Study of Client Perceptions of Traumatic Incident Reduction (TIR): a Brief Trauma Treatment." *Crisis Intervention and Time-Limited Treatment,* v. 4, no. 1, pp. 1-12, 1998, ISSN: 1064-5136

Valentine, P. "Traumatic Incident Reduction: A Review of a New Intervention." *Journal of Family Psychotherapy,* 6, (2), 79-85, 1995.

Whitfield, H. (2006). Towards case-specific applications of mindfulness-based cognitive-behavioural therapies: a mindfulness-based rational emotive behaviour therapy . *Counselling Psy-chology Quarterly, 19*(2), 205-218.

Wylie, M. S. "Researching PTSD: Going for the Cure." *Family Therapy Networker*, 20(4), pp. 20-37, July/Aug. 1996.

Annotated Bibliography

Figley, C. (2002). *Brief Treatments for the Traumatized: A Project of the Green Cross Foundation*, CRC Press, ISBN: 031332137X, pp. 252-265 (Chapter 12 by Pamela Vest Valentine, Ph.D. on TIR)

Cooper, C. (2002). *Bullying and Emotional Abuse in the Workplace: International Perspectives in Research and Practice.* ISBN 0415253594, CRC Press, 2002. (p. 276 article by Noreen Te-hrani "Illustrates how TIR help a manager deal with the painful memory of a difficult team meeting." with actual session dialog.)

Ecker, B. and Hulley, L. (1995) *Depth Oriented Brief Therapy (DOBT) : How to Be Brief When You Were Trained to Be Deep and Vice Versa* " Jossey-Bass Social and Behavioral Science Series) ISBN: 0787901520. (p. 217: "In DOBT terms, the TIR technique efficiently carries out radical inquiry and position work in rela-tion to a particular type of pro-symptom position, one in which the (ongoing) emotional reality was formed by a traumatic inci-dent. This repetitive, detailed, subjective review instigates a thorough emotional processing of this memory, progressively filling in lost details and unfolding the crucial moments of meaning-formation that occurred during the incident. This brings about a spontaneous emergence into awareness of the symptom-generating meanings, construals, intentions, and pro-tective actions that were unconsciously formed. Thus, the TIR process fits very well within the DOBT framework of psychothe-rapy.")

Dryden, W. and Neenan, M. (2005). *Counselling Individuals: A Ra-tional Emotive Behavioural Handbook, 4th Ed.* by. (Mentions that TIR is effective for PTSD symptoms.)

Gold, S.L. (2000) *Not Trauma Alone: Therapy for Child Abuse Survi-vors in Family and Social Context*, ISBN: 1583910271, Brunner-Routledge. (pp. 220-227 recommends TIR for use with survivors of PCA [Prolonged Child Abuse]).

Harris, C.J. in *Simple and Complex Post-Traumatic Stress Disorder: Strategies for Comprehensive Treatment in Clinical Practice* (2002) by Mary Beth Williams ISBN: 0789002981, Haworth

Press. (Chapter 12. p. 270 "Using TIR as the treatment of choice for the family members when there is vicarious, chiasmal, or intra-family trauma should allow the family therapist to treat the individual family members in a relatively brief time.")

Oz, Sheri (2005). "The Wall of Fear: The Bridge Between the Traumatic Event and Trauma Resolution Therapy for Childhood Sexual Abuse Survivors" in *Journal of Child Sexual Abuse* Ed. by Eitan, M and Motzkin, K. ISSN: 1053-8712 14:3.

Roberts, A.R. (2000). *Crisis Intervention Handbook: Assessment, Treatment, and Research* Ed, ISBN: 019513365X, Oxford University Press. (chapter by Pamela Vest Valentine, Ph.D. on Adult Survivors of Incest: p. 265 states that "Both TIR and group treatment have been tested and found effective in assisting clients in answering old questions and generating new options."

Roberts, C.A. (2003.) *Coping with Post-Traumatic Stress Disorder: A Guide for Families*, by Cheryl A. Roberts, McFarland & Company, 2003 ISBN 0786417366 , pp. 96-97 (Chapter 7 discusses EMDR and TIR)

Spiers, T. (2002). *Trauma: A Practitioners Guide to Counselling*. ISBN: 0415186943. Brunner-Routledge. (p. 119 says that "Clients who have a tendency to cut off from their feelings when talking about the incident may benefit from TIR" There are a few other mentions throughout the book.

Tudor, K. (2008). *Brief Person-Centered Therapies*. ISBN: 9781847873477. Article by Henry Whitfield: "Traumatic Incident Reduction and Applied Metapsychology Techniques: Operationalising Rogerian Theory in a Brief Therapy Practice." Explains how TIR can be both therapist-directed and still claim to operate in the Rogerian (undirected) regime.

Williams, M.B. and Nurmi, L.A. (2001) *Creating a Comprehensive Trauma Center: Choices and Challenges*. ISBN 030646327X, Plenum Press. (p. 38 indicates that "TIR may be effective for uncomplicated PTSD."

Wolfe, A.T. (2005) *Got Parts? An Insider's Guide to Managing Life Successfully with Dissociative Identity Disorder*, ISBN 1932690034. Ann Arbor: Loving Healing Press (p. 170 mentions TIR for use with adult Dissociative Identity Disorder clients)

Index

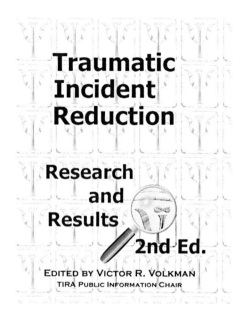

Traumatic Incident Reduction

Research and Results
2nd Ed.

EDITED BY VICTOR R. VOLKMAN
TIRA PUBLIC INFORMATION CHAIR

Traumatic Incident Reduction: Research & Results provides synopses of several TIR research projects from the early 1990s to the very latest. Each article, in the researcher's own words, provides new insights into the effectiveness of Traumatic Incident Reduction. The three doctoral dissertation level studies that form the core of this book investigate the outcome results of TIR with crime victims, incarcerated females, and anxiety and panic disorders respectively (Bisbey, Valentine, and Coughlin.)

Both informal and formal reports of the "Active Ingredient" study by Charles R. Figley and Joyce Carbonell of Florida State University investigate how TIR and other brief treatments for traumatic stress provide relief. A further case study by Teresa Descilo, MSW informs of outcomes from an ongoing project to provide help to at-risk middle-school students in an inner-city setting.

An introduction by Robert H. Moore, Ph.D. provides background into how TIR provides relief for symptoms of Post-Traumatic Stress Disorder (PTSD) and firmly establishes the roots of TIR in the traditions of desensitization, imaginal flooding, and Rogerian techniques.

ISBN 978-1-932690-50-7   **$24.95**

WWW.TIRBOOK.COM
TO ORDER: 888-761-6268